# The Holistic Body

## A Guide to Embracing a
## Simply Holistic Lifestyle

By
Stephanie Seborg,
LMT, Healer & Spiritual Guide
&
Sharry Smith,
LMT & Holistic Lifestyle Guide

ISBN: 979-8-9891941-4-8 (paperback)
ISBN:  979-8-9891941-8-6 (e-book)

This book is dedicated to our families and friends who have supported us throughout our healing. The teachers, mentors, and guides that have helped us learn and grow within our strengths. All those whom we have been blessed to help find their healing path. And all those who are yet to come. We bless you all with peace and good health.

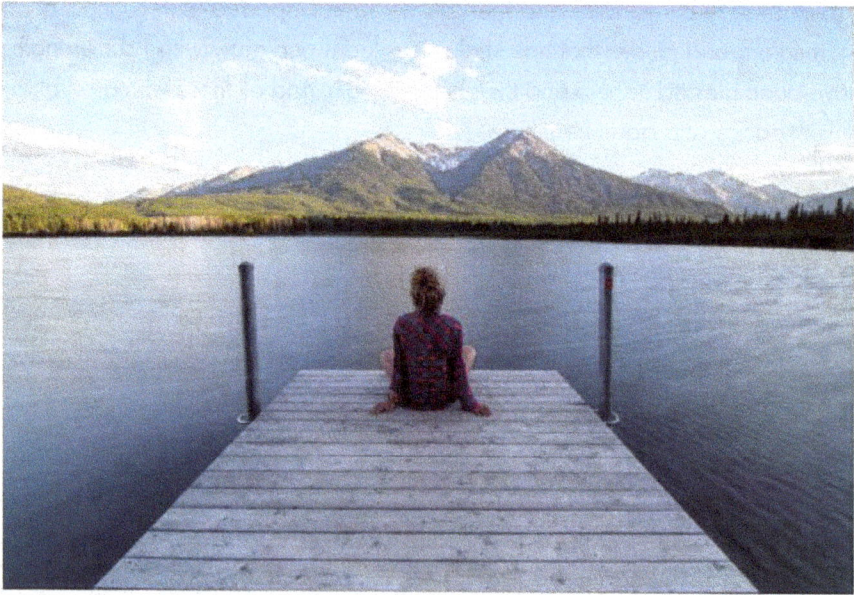

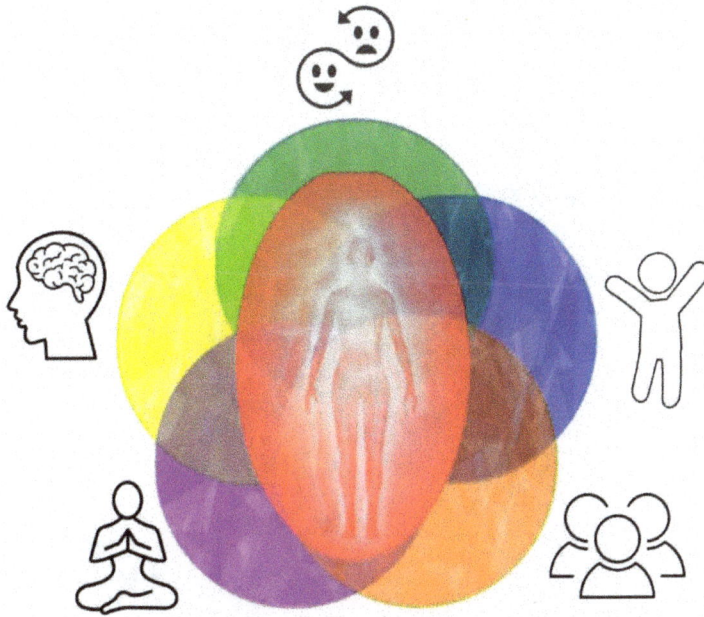

# The Holistic Body

A Guide to Embracing a
Simply Holistic Lifestyle

# Contents

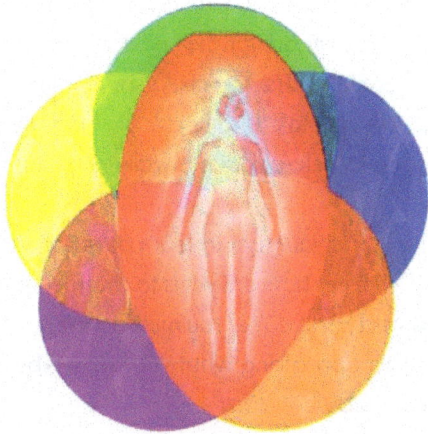

## Introduction

Congratulations! You have begun your wellness journey and found an excellent resource for learning the holistic approach to restoring and maintaining optimal health. With the information you gain from *The Holistic Body*, you will be able to address health issues you may be having or want to avoid.

Embracing a holistic lifestyle involves conscious and deliberate physical, mental, emotional, social, and spiritual health choices. It means prioritizing the natural and organic over the synthetic and focusing on sustainable practices that support your overall well-being.

There is no one-size-fits-all approach to living a holistic lifestyle. Still, some standard methods include eating whole, nutritious foods, engaging in regular physical activity, self-care, connecting with nature, and prioritizing relationships and community.

This book will give you the information to start your journey to a holistic body. We recommend that you use this book along with a journal to document this life-changing journey to reflect on the fantastic changes that manifest for you.

Let's take a quick inventory. Are you feeling completely balanced and harmonious in your mental state right now? How about your emotional state? Your physical state? Your social state? And, finally, your spiritual condition?

Most of us will have a few areas that need work to find that balance and reach a healthy state. Do you suffer from mental issues like depression, anxiety, ADD, or Bipolar Disorder? Are you a person who struggles to think positive thoughts continuously? Believe us when we say if you suffer from mental or emotional imbalances, you most likely feel them in your physical, social, and even spiritual life.

Do you often break down from the pressures of life? We all know how it feels to be under pressure in our environment. Home, work, driving, or social events can trigger emotional, mental, social, physical, and spiritual discomfort. Often, we feel this as pain. Do you suffer from chronic physical, mental, emotional, social, or spiritual distress? What does this look like? Noticing and being mindful of how life pressures affect your health and well-being is a start on the road to wellness.

What do we mean by embracing a holistic yet simple lifestyle?

First, to live a life of simplicity has its health benefits. Some of the benefits of living a simple life include:

- More time for what matters most

- Less stress and more relaxation
- Increased mental clarity and focus
- Improved physical and emotional health
- Better sleep quality
- More financial independence and stability
- Stronger relationships with family and friends
- Increased creativity and productivity
- Greater appreciation for the little things in life
- Reduced environmental impact and greater sustainability.

Living a simple life can help you achieve balance, peace, and harmony. Who wouldn't want to have most of the listed benefits above? It takes just a few adjustments to your daily routine to create a simple and holistic life, which leads to optimal health.

We, the authors, have spent many years learning, practicing, and integrating holistic practices into our lives. We have both overcome disabilities that mainstream medical professionals said were impossible! We were told that we would never get better and that we just had to take our prescription drugs and live with the disabilities.

Being the strong, independent women that we are, we said, "You don't know us very well!" to those doctors. Once we decided that there had to be another way, a way that didn't involve taking medications for the rest of our lives. That is when we dove deep into learning all of the holistic, alternative, complementary, and integrative approaches to getting well. Our years of study and practice paid off, not just for our health but for the health of many clients over the years. You could say that we strive to live a simple and holistic life and use our knowledge to help our clients walk the holistic path.

Now, it is your turn to learn or reacquaint yourself with just how easy it is to change your lifestyle and health. Yes, you must do the work — learning and practicing what you know — but the rewards will be bountiful!

Take a moment to close your eyes and see yourself in your mind. Picture yourself in your healthiest and most vibrant state. What does being unencumbered and free of health issues look like? Make a note about how you feel — do you see physical and mental strength and flexibility? Emotional stamina and integrity? Spiritual calm and peace? Visualizing yourself in your healthiest and most balanced state is a powerful tool to keep you on track to achieving optimal health.

In this book, you will gain the knowledge you need to begin a simple and holistic life, leading you to that healthy and vibrant picture you created of yourself. You will also find easy-to-follow instructions to start practicing your learning in each section. We have done our best to provide you with great information and the tools you need to start your path to a holistic body. Take your time to soak in the information and take action by doing something every day to practice what you learn.

Journal and pen in hand, let's begin.

## Take a Moment

_____

_____

_____

_____

_____

_____

_____

_____

_____

_____

_____

_____

_____

_____

_____

_____

_____

_____

_____

_____

_____

_____

_____

_____

_____

_____

_____

_____

_____

_____

_____

_____

_____

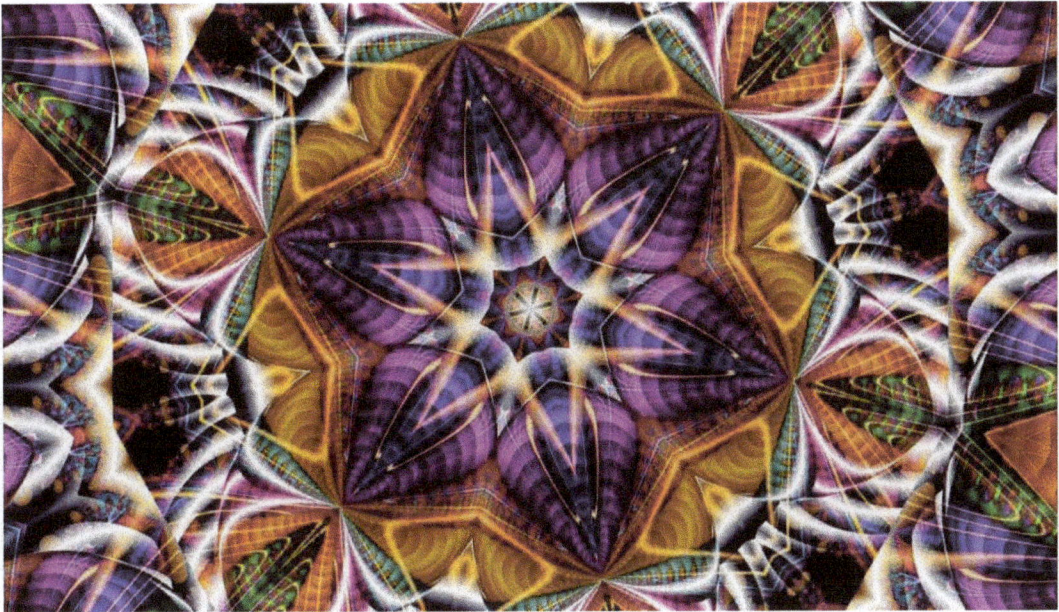

# PART I: The Holistic Body

Part I lays the foundation for *The Holistic Body: A Guide to Embracing a Simply Holistic Lifestyle* by exploring Holistic Health and how it can improve individual health.

- Characteristics of Holistic Health
- The history of Holistic Health
- What is the purpose of Holistic Health?
- How can I bring Holistic Health practices into my daily life?
- How do I find a Holistic Health professional to help me?

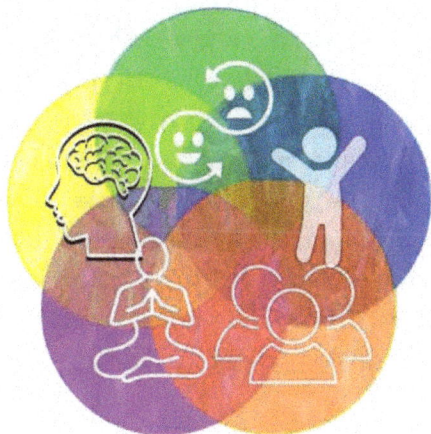

# Chapter One: Foundations of Holistic Health

*"Wellness encompasses a healthy body, a sound mind, and a tranquil spirit. Enjoy the journey as you strive for wellness."*
-Laurette Gagnon Beaulieu

## Characteristics of Holistic Health

Holistic health is an approach to wellness that considers the whole person, including their physical, mental, emotional, social, and spiritual well-being, rather than just focusing on a specific illness or symptom. It is based on the idea that each aspect of a person's life is interconnected and that addressing all areas of life can lead to optimal health and well-being. This approach to health and healing incorporates a variety of natural and alternative therapies and traditional medical treatments. It is about integration. People who practice holistic health believe that

by bringing the body, mind, and spirit into balance, individuals can achieve optimal health and wellness.

Holistic health incorporates all aspects of well-being, including physical, mental, emotional, social, and spiritual health. By considering the interconnectedness of these areas, holistic health practitioners can develop a personalized health plan that supports the person's overall well-being. For example, exercise and healthy eating can improve physical health, while mindfulness and relaxation techniques can help mental and emotional health. Social connection and engagement in enjoyable activities can support a person's social and emotional well-being. By treating the whole person rather than just focusing on a specific symptom or illness, holistic health practices support overall health and well-being and can help prevent future health problems.

One way holistic health practices promote prevention is by focusing on healthy eating habits and regular physical activity, which can help lower the risk of many chronic diseases, such as heart disease and diabetes. Other practices, such as meditation and stress management techniques, can help reduce the risk of hormone imbalances and lower blood pressure.

Holistic health practitioners also focus on preventive measures such as regular check-ups and screenings to detect health problems early when they are most treatable. By taking a proactive approach to health and wellness, holistic health can help prevent many common health problems and provide tools for awareness of irregularities in the body.

Multidimensional aspects of well-being are considered in holistic health because what affects one part of well-being affects others. Consider that an injury to the body also impacts emotional and mental wellness and can even affect other areas of the body. Some of the aspects include:

- Recognition of the whole person: Holistic health focuses on treating the individual, including physical, emotional, mental, and spiritual aspects.
- Integration of therapies: Holistic health integrates natural and conventional therapies, including alternative therapies like acupuncture, yoga, and meditation, alongside traditional medical treatments.
- Prevention: Holistic health emphasizes the importance of prevention, early detection, and treatment of illnesses and diseases.
- Personalization: Holistic health recognizes that each person is unique and tailors treatments to individual needs and preferences.
- Mind-body connection: Holistic health emphasizes the interconnectedness of the mind and body and recognizes mental and emotional health's impact on physical fitness and vice versa.
- Healthy lifestyle practices: Holistic health encourages individuals to adopt healthy lifestyles, including a nutritious diet, regular exercise, and stress management techniques.
- Spiritual health: Holistic health recognizes that spiritual health is an essential aspect of

overall well-being and encourages individuals to connect with their spirituality through practices like prayer, meditation, or mindfulness.

Holistic health recognizes that individual health is not just dependent on the physical body but is a result of multiple factors contributing to well-being and vitality.

We have used many of these approaches to reach our health goals. Our lives prove that bumps in the road exist regarding health. Like us, you can go through holistic health resources to find what is needed and turn them into tools to overcome new challenges.

## A Brief History of Holistic Health

Healers and practitioners throughout history have incorporated natural remedies and therapies into their practices. Ancient healers, well before the advent of modern medicine, developed holistic health practices even before the documented methods of Ayurveda and Traditional Chinese Medicine. Even Hippocrates, the father of modern clinical medicine, recognized the healing powers of nature and the body's ability to self-heal in the 4th century BCE. Although Western holistic practices began in ancient Greece, the modern holistic movement started in the late 1960s. People thought modern medicine focused too much on drugs and medical technology and instead believed in treating the whole person, including their emotional, social, and spiritual well-being.

Modern nursing has been grounded in holistic principles since the 1700s, using natural remedies and healing therapies alongside conventional medicine.

The use of complementary and alternative medicine has grown in popularity over the years, with practices such as acupuncture, herbal medicine, and energy healing.

We feel honored to be able to use, and help others use, the tools that holistic health offers. We have both done research on ancient healing traditions and modern healing techniques, which we have brought into our daily practice. We feel equally honored to share some of this information with you as you strive to reach your health goals.

## Identifying How Holistic Health Can Help You

Researching holistic health involves exploring a variety of resources, including government agencies, research institutions, professional organizations, and peer-reviewed journals. The Holistic Body is a great foundation to begin your exploration.

The first step is to try holistic approaches that call to you. There are a variety of holistic, alternative, and complementary approaches out there. As you research, find and note some of the techniques or ideas you desire to try out, record the experience in your journal, and see if you are called to try it again. Remember that some approaches and modalities may feel incomplete at first. Reiki or energy work, for example, is so subtle that you may not be immediately aware of any results in the first round of trying it. So, don't give up on many approaches after the first round. Try again and follow what your inner guidance is telling you!

Secondly, you can research modalities and find guidance from professionals. There are many holistic practitioners to choose from online or in your community. Even small communities have their natural healers. No matter where you live, you can find a professional to work with you. If you have access to the internet, then your options are limitless.

Some examples of holistic professionals include:

- Holistic Health Practitioners, Coaches, or Guides
- Naturopathic Doctors
- Acupuncturists
- Chiropractors
- Homeopaths
- Massage Therapists
- Energy Healers (such as Reiki or Pranic Healing practitioners)
- Ayurvedic Practitioners
- Holistic Nutritionists or Dietitians
- Traditional Chinese Medicine Practitioners

These professionals take a holistic approach to their work, focusing on the whole person and considering health and wellness's physical, emotional, mental, and spiritual aspects. They may use a variety of natural healing and therapeutic methods to promote healing and well-being.

Third, research holistic health in general. Some essential resources to consider:

- National Center for Complementary and Integrative Health (NCCIH) - This government organization provides research on complementary and alternative medicine and holistic health practices.
- Academy of Natural Health Sciences - This academic institution researches alternative and holistic health practices.

- Natural Medicines Comprehensive Database - This database provides information on herbal supplements and other natural products commonly used in holistic health practices.
- Mayo Clinic - The Mayo Clinic provides information on integrative medicine and holistic health, including research on their effectiveness.
- Journals - Several peer-reviewed journals publish research on holistic health practices. Some examples include the Journal of Holistic Nursing, Explore: The Journal of Science and Healing, and the Journal of Alternative and Complementary Medicine.

Finally, listen to your body. While researching is essential, also be sure to listen to your body to see if the modality, practice, or food agrees with you. If you try yoga and are not quite ready for that level of physical or mental challenge, start with something more manageable, like Qigong or walking in nature. A remedy, food, or activity that makes some people feel wonderful may not resonate with others. No matter what a professional tells you or the hype surrounding a particular product or diet, only your body can tell whether the modality, practice, or treatment works for you. You know your body more than anyone else, so trust your body and instincts.

## The Starfish Story (Adapted from the original story by Lauren Eisley)

Once upon a time, there was an elder who used to go to the seaside every morning to write. They had a habit of walking along the beautiful beach before starting their work. One beautiful day, as per the morning ritual, they went to the seashore and started walking. After some time, they came along a stretch upon which thousands of starfish had been stranded. The beach was littered with starfish as far as the eye could see, stretching in both directions!

Off in the distance, the old one noticed a little child approaching. As the child walked, they paused occasionally, bending down to pick up an object and throw it into the sea.

The young one came closer, and the ancient called, "Good morning, little one!!! May I ask what it is that you are doing?" The child paused, looked up, and replied, "Throwing starfish into the sea." Then, the child continued picking up and throwing the starfish back into the sea.

"I must ask, why are you throwing starfish into the sea?"

The little child replied "The tide has washed them onto the beach, and they can't return to the sea alone. Unless I throw them back into the water, they will die when the sun gets high." Upon hearing this, the ancient one commented, "But, child, do you not realize that there are miles and miles of beach and starfish all along every mile? There must be tens of thousands of starfish on this beach. I'm afraid you won't be able to make much of a difference."

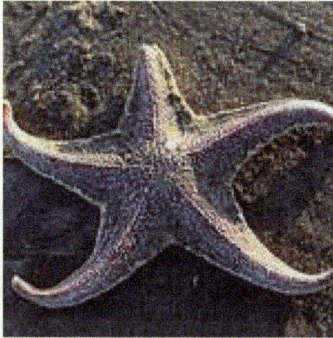

Image by L'Oriol.

The wise child bent down, picked up yet another starfish, and threw it into the ocean as far as they could. Then, turning towards the old one, smiled sweetly, and said, *"I made a difference to that one!"*

Gracefully acknowledging that truth, the old one began to help save starfish that day.

In life, we get several opportunities to create positive change, but we often need more time and wait for someone, anyone, else to do something. We avoid the more significant challenges by rationalizing, "How much of a difference can I make?" You might not be able to change the whole world, but at least you can change a small part. Be the change for yourself.

The child teaches us that we should never surrender hope, no matter how complex the challenges or situations are. The child lives with hope in something unknowable and believes in trying and making an effort to make a difference. Their life is more meaningful because they live with hope and inspire others with their actions.

## Key Takeaways

Holistic health is an approach to wellness that considers the whole person, including their physical, mental, emotional, social, and spiritual well-being. By addressing all aspects of a person's well-being and promoting healthy habits and lifestyles, holistic health practitioners believe they can help prevent many common health problems and promote overall wellness.

### Characteristics of holistic health include:
- Recognition of the whole person
- Integration of therapies
- Prevention
- Personalization
- Mind-body connection
- Healthy lifestyle practices
- Spiritual health

### Holistic health has many benefits, including:
- Addresses the whole person
- Identifies underlying causes
- Encourages healthy lifestyle
- Personalized attention
- Use of natural resources and methods
- Stress reduction

### Where do you start?
- Try Holistic Approaches That Call to You
- Find Guidance from a Professional
- Do Research
- Listen to Your Body

## Questions For Reflection:

1. **What holistic resources do I currently use?**
2. **What are my health goals now?**
3. **What holistic practitioners have I seen lately?**
4. **Which holistic practitioners would I like to see?**

*Take a Moment*

_____
_____
_____
_____
_____
_____
_____
_____
_____
_____
_____
_____
_____
_____

There is a surge of people who are disenchanted with mainstream doctors and healthcare. They are looking for holistic and integrative approaches to fill in the gaps they feel in their healthcare. In the next chapter, you will learn the whys and what makes holistic health so popular.

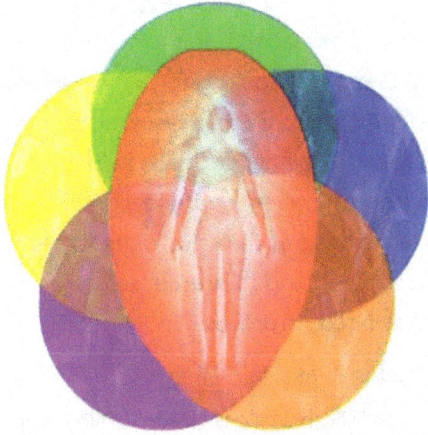

# Chapter Two: Holistic Health

"Wellness is not a 'medical fix' but a way of living —
a lifestyle sensitive and responsive to all the
dimensions of body, mind, spirit, an approach to life
we each design to achieve our highest potential for
well-being now and forever."
-Greg Anderson

## Why Has Holistic Health Become So Popular?

Holistic health is becoming more popular because it offers a way to address all aspects of a person's health and well-being. Many people seek natural ways to promote their overall health and well-being, and holistic health practices often offer a way to do this without relying on medication or other conventional medical treatments. As a result, many people are turning to holistic health practices to take a more proactive approach to their health and well-being.

Holistic health work empowers people to take their health into their own hands, which is vital to genuinely making a difference in health and mental outlook. After all, you are the one who knows you the best. When you are self-empowered, you are in control of your own life and can achieve health benefits that may include:

- Mood boost: Regular exercise and eating healthy meals can boost your mood and mental health.
- Higher self-esteem: Self-empowerment can lead to higher self-esteem and lower chances of experiencing mental health conditions like depression or anxiety.
- Reduced stress: Empowerment can give you a feeling of control and reduce stress, which can positively impact your physical and mental health.
- Self-care: Empowering yourself can help promote self-care, which requires being kind and caring for your physical and mental health.

## What Are the Most Popular Holistic Therapies?

The most popular holistic therapies include:

- Reflexology: a therapy that involves applying pressure to specific points on the feet, hands, or ears to promote healing and relaxation.
- Massage therapy: a therapy that involves manipulating soft tissues to promote relaxation and relieve muscle tension.
- Acupuncture: a therapy that involves inserting needles at specific points on the

body to stimulate energy flow and promote healing.

- Yoga: a therapy that involves physical postures, breathing exercises, and meditation to promote health and well-being.
- Aromatherapy: a therapy that uses essential oils for their therapeutic properties, such as calming the mind and promoting relaxation.
- Chiropractic: a therapy that involves manipulating the spine to correct alignment and improve overall health and well-being.

Other popular holistic therapies, such as meditation, tai chi, and reiki, can also benefit the body and overall well-being. The popularity of these therapies vary by region and individual preferences. Fortunately, there are many therapies and modalities from which to choose! You may even find that your priorities and preferred modalities change over time.

## What Is Holistic Coaching?

Holistic coaching is a type of coaching that takes a comprehensive approach to an individual's life and well-being. Holistic coaches work with clients to identify areas of their lives that may be causing stress, imbalance, or dissatisfaction and help them set goals and develop plans to achieve more outstanding balance and fulfillment. Holistic coaches may draw from various techniques and practices, such as mindfulness, meditation, visualization, and energy work, to help clients achieve their goals and improve their overall quality of life. Holistic health coaching empowers individuals to make lasting changes to enhance health and well-being.

Finding the right coach can be particularly beneficial for individuals who have struggled to achieve their health goals using traditional medicine or are looking for a more integrated and holistic approach to their health and wellness. A Holistic coach can help individuals develop a greater awareness and understanding of their bodies, thoughts, and emotions, leading to greater self-awareness and self-care practices.

## What Is a Holistic Lifestyle?

A holistic lifestyle is a way of life that emphasizes the interconnectedness of physical, mental, emotional, social, and spiritual health. It involves taking a comprehensive approach to one's well-being rather than focusing on isolated areas of health or wellness. A holistic lifestyle often involves healthy eating habits, regular exercise, stress management techniques, and mindfulness or meditation. Living a holistic lifestyle aims to achieve overall balance and harmony between different areas of your life.

Here are some holistic lifestyle tips that can help you improve your holistic being:

- Practice mindfulness: Taking a few minutes each day to focus on the present moment can be very beneficial for reducing stress and improving mental clarity. As you focus on your environment and senses, you may also become aware of unrecognized interference to your peace.
- Practice meditation: Achieving inner peace and relaxation is helpful for not only improving one's emotions and mindset but also has physical and spiritual benefits. Whether you focus on your breathing or

listen to a guided meditation, this practice's help is plentiful and increases over time.

- Eat a healthy diet: Eating whole, unprocessed foods and avoiding excess sugar, salt, and unhealthy fats can help you maintain a healthy weight and reduce your risk of heart disease, type 2 diabetes, stroke, and certain cancers. A healthy diet that includes omega-3 fatty acids, antioxidants, and vitamins and minerals supports brain health, which can improve memory and concentration.

- Incorporate regular exercise: Regular physical activity can help improve physical health, reduce stress, and boost mood as well as helping to achieve and maintain a healthy weight, build a strong body and heart, and increase energy levels.

- Get enough restful sleep: Adequate sleep is essential for overall health and well-being. Aim for 7-8 hours of quality sleep each night to improve cognitive function, enhance mood, boost the immune system, and improve physical and mental performance.

- Incorporate self-care practices: Taking time to do things you enjoy, such as relaxing or getting a massage, can help reduce stress and promote overall well-being. Regular self-care techniques can enhance overall resilience, which, in turn, can help you better cope with stressors and maintain a positive outlook during difficult times.

- Stay connected with loved ones: Maintaining close relationships with friends and family is essential for social support, which can help reduce the risk of mental health issues. Social interactions and emotional support from loved ones can help you feel more secure, validated, and understood, contributing to a better outlook on life.

- Incorporate spiritual health: This can include things like meditation, yoga, or connecting with nature and the world around you. Spiritual exercises can help you connect with something greater than yourself and help you find meaning and a purpose in life. Spiritual beliefs and practices can provide comfort, hope, and strength during difficult times.

- Natural remedies: Incorporate natural therapies, such as herbal teas or aromatherapy, into your routine to support physical and emotional health. Natural remedies often have fewer side effects than conventional medicine. However, it's important to note that natural remedies can still interact with other medications, so it's essential to consult your doctor and herbalist before taking anything new.

Remember that a holistic approach to health and well-being involves creating balance and harmony in all areas of your life, not just focusing on one aspect in isolation. Many people who get hyper-focused on one aspect of health or another, such as those who get obsessed with physical exercise and have a daily routine that can last for hours or those who are so overwhelmed with their emotional state that they think they should focus on only one thing to fix it (usually mental health counseling). Holistic healing and work allow the e compasses physical, emotional, mental, spiritual, and social health.

You can support your overall health by incorporating holistic lifestyle practices into your daily routine. These are things that you can do on your own to get started. The key is not just to try one, but to try them ALL! Don't make it complicated, though. Keeping it simple makes it less confusing and disruptive to our lives. Embracing a simple and holistic lifestyle is all about taking what you have learned about holistic practices and slowly starting to incorporate them and see how they work for you in your daily life.

## Finding a Holistic Health Professional

There are several resources you can use to find a holistic health practitioner:

- Ask for recommendations from family and friends with experience working with holistic health practitioners.
- Check with your insurance company to see if they cover visits to holistic health practitioners and get a list of covered providers.
- Check with local holistic health organizations or associations to see if they can provide recommendations or referrals.
- Use online directories, such as the American Holistic Medical Association website or the Holistic Health Directory, to search for practitioners in your area.
- Consider using the "Find a Practitioner" tool on the Institute for Functional Medicine website to search for functional medicine practitioners in your area.
- Use Holistic Bodyworks Online resources to find holistic professionals and products that you can use from the comfort of your home.

You can find a holistic health practitioner who aligns with your needs and preferences and supports your holistic health goals using these resources. But, just like anything you do on your path to health and wellness, follow what your body, mind, and spirit are telling you. In other words, YOU get to pick who and what works for you. If you don't feel comfortable with one professional, or practice, choose another.

## Key Takeaways

Holistic health is becoming more popular because it offers a way to address all aspects of a person's health and well-being and exponentially increase one's self-empowerment and enjoyment of life. Many people seek natural ways to promote their overall health and well-being, and holistic health practices often offer a way to do this without relying on medication or other conventional medical treatments.

We have helped many clients over the years who have reached a point in their health where they are fed up with the conventional treatments their regular doctor is doing for them. They are tired of being on the medications that cause side effects and being told by their doctor that nothing else can be done. Hearing words like, "It's all in your head," "You'll have to stay on this medication for the rest of your life," and "All of the tests show that there is nothing wrong with you" can put a damper on how you feel about your health. This is where having a great holistic coach or professional can be so empowering. You do not need to take those medications forever!

If you get to a state of homeostasis, then you won't need the medicine anymore. If you are told nothing is wrong because it doesn't show up on the tests, that doesn't mean there isn't an imbalance that can be found and fixed!

With the right professional, you can start feeling what self-empowerment can do for your health. You can begin to find the right combination of practices that will be perfect to bring yourself into harmony and balance. You have the power to improve your health and he right professional will teach and guide you to do it yourself!

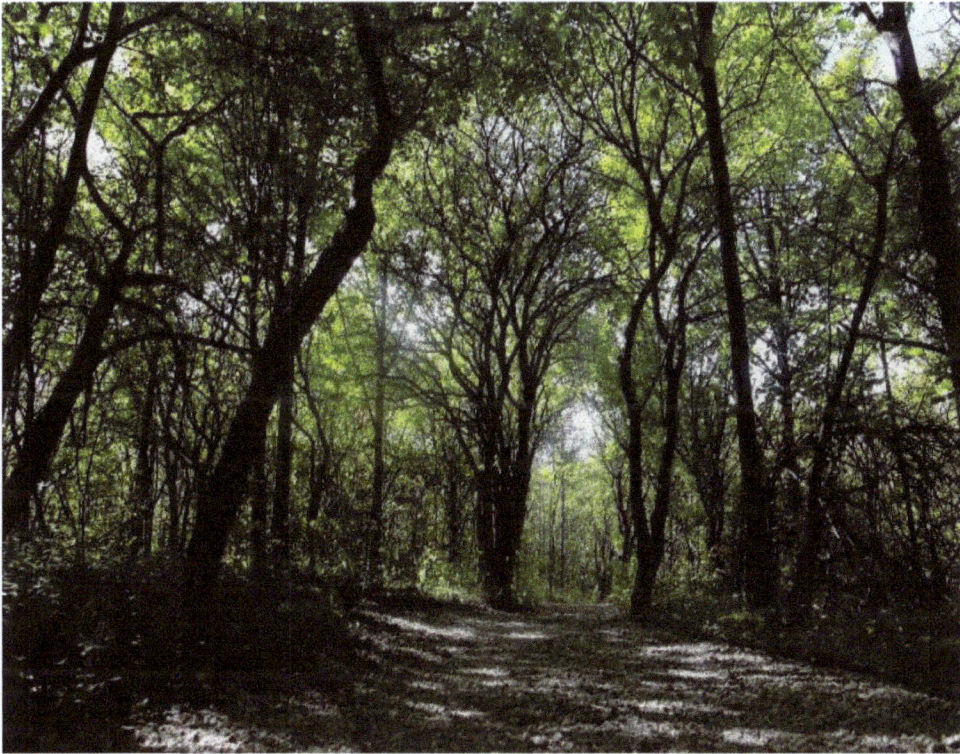
Image by Atraktor Studio

## Questions For Reflection:

1. Which popular holistic modalities have I tried already?
2. Which holistic modalities would I like to try?
3. How can I bring holistic self-care into my daily life?

*Take a Moment*

_____

_____

_____

_____

_____

_____

_____

_____

_____

_____

_____

_____

_____

_____

In the next chapter, you will dive into the physical aspects of holistic health, the importance of working on your physical health, and how to bring physical elements into your routine. It's time to get into the 'meat' of your physical health and bring some holistic practices into your life!

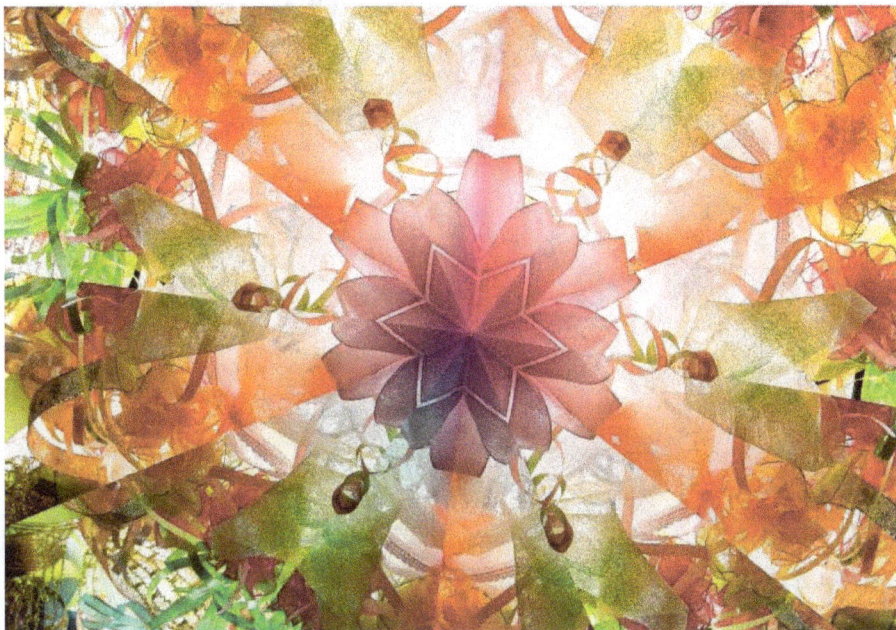

# PART II: 5 Aspects of Holistic Health

Part II explores the five aspects of holistic health and how you can bring each aspect into your daily life.

- Physical Aspects of Holistic Health
- Mental Aspects of Holistic Health
- Social Aspects of Holistic Health
- Spiritual Aspects of Holistic Health
- Emotional Aspects of Holistic Health

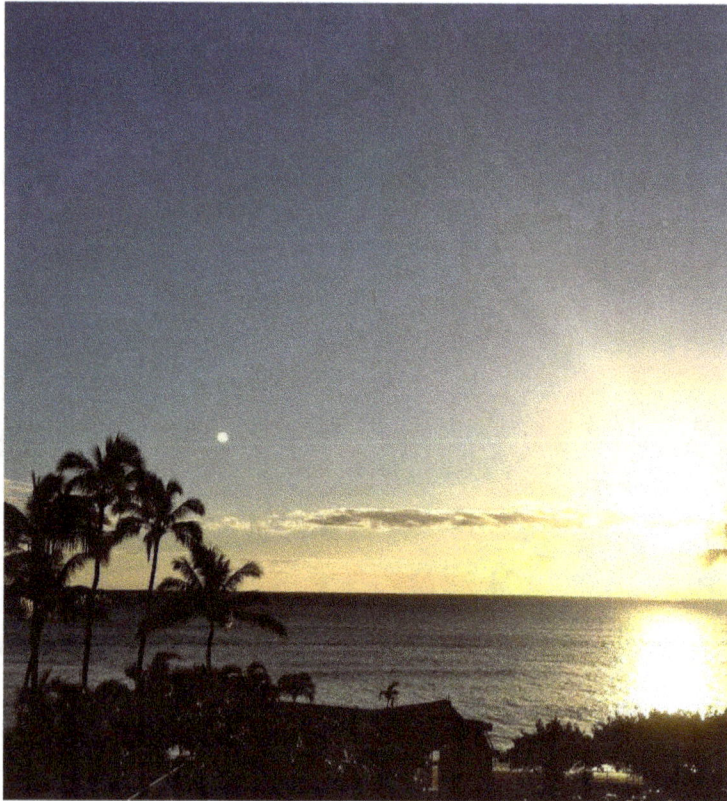

Image by Liesl Seborg

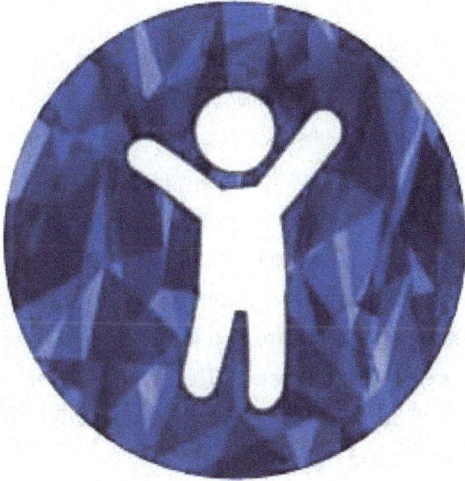

# Chapter Three: Physical Aspects of Holistic Health

*"Our bodies are our gardens –*
*our wills are our gardeners."*
*-William Shakespeare*

## Why is Physical Health Important?

Physical health is a crucial component of overall health and vitality. Regular physical activity can help maintain healthy weight, strengthen bones and muscles, reduce the risk of chronic diseases (such as diabetes, heart disease, and stroke), and improve cardiovascular and respiratory health. In addition to these physical benefits, regular physical activity positively affects mental health, including reducing feelings of anxiety and depression, improving mood, and reducing stress levels. Adequate sleep and a healthy diet also contribute to physical health.

Physical health and vitality are essential to leading a fulfilling and meaningful life. When a person is in good physical health, they have the energy to confidently engage in daily activities and pursue their goals and interests. A healthy body helps promote self-esteem and positive body image, which can profoundly impact mental health and overall well-being.

Individuals are the world are taking essential steps toward ensuring their overall quality of life by prioritizing physical health through regular exercise, a nutritious diet, and adequate sleep.

How is your physical health? Do you feel physically fit and healthy? If not, you may need to bring more of the physical aspect of holistic health into your life. You don't need to go to the gym - you can go for a nice walk or do some yoga in the park. As with everything, you can choose what works for you. You can pick up a new and fun physical activity like roller skating, jump rope, or kick boxing. Get creative and make it fun!

Whether a person can be overweight and still be healthy is a topic of debate right now because, generally, excess weight is associated with an increased risk of health issues, such as diabetes, heart disease, and high blood pressure. However, some individuals are classified as overweight and have good overall health. It is essential to note that this is uncommon and that most overweight people experience adverse health effects.

One thing we all have in common is that we are all living in physical human bodies. We come in different sizes, shapes, colors and abilities. Some of us have been here briefly, and others have been here for decades. We all need to eat, drink, and sleep. We all need shelter. Those are the necessities for humans to live.

Our bodies were designed to move. There are over 200 joints and muscles in our human body, and those joints and muscles all work together so we can walk, run, reach, lift, climb stairs, and do whatever else we need or want to do during our day. If we keep those joints and muscles in good working order, we can move freely all our lives. We may slow down some, but we will be able to care for ourselves and each other.

When we don't keep our bodies moving, stiffness and soreness set in and limit our abilities. This is often attributed to aging, but in many cases, it is simply a lack of movement that, over time, has reduced our capabilities. When our muscles aren't used, they atrophy and may forget how to properly function.

Another thing we need to stay moving is good nutrition. Vitamins, minerals, healthy fats, and fiber are essential to provide our joints and muscles the energy they need to keep moving. Fresh fruit and vegetables, lean meat and fish, seeds, and nuts are what our body was designed to use and create this energy.

Sometimes, illness or injury will occur. This is just part of life. We can avoid damage by practicing safety measures, such as wearing a seat belt in a car, having someone help you lift something heavy, and things of that nature. We can avoid some illnesses by eating healthy food, drinking plenty of clean water, and avoiding cigarettes and excessive alcohol or drugs.

There is no guarantee in life that illness or injury will never happen. If and when it does, we can recover better and faster if we are already healthy. Science has discovered that if we need medication or surgery, the medical intervention works better in a systemically sound body at the onset.

Our bodies were designed with a built-in healing mechanism, and it works well when it receives what it needs. Think of how a cut heals after a few days or we get over a cold. That's the healing mechanism at work. But the healing mechanism may also become weak when our body is depleted of necessary vitamins and minerals from poor dietary choices or if we have been sedentary for prolonged periods.

Movement is medicine. Movement generates chemicals in our bloodstream that our healing mechanism needs. Movement helps our body to rid itself of toxins, cellular debris, and undigested food that need to be discarded. Without movement, this debris can build up and become toxic to us, causing disease and other uncomfortable health situations.

A healthy diet and regular movement can lead to better recoveries from illness and injury and help us enjoy feeling good all our lives. No matter what state of health you are in, no matter your age, there is always time to make changes.

## PHYSICAL HEALTH FIRST STEPS

- GET REGULAR EXERCISE
- GIVE YOUR BODY PROPER NUTRITION
- GET REGULAR MEDICAL CHECK-UPS AND SCREENINGS
- FOLLOW PREVENTATIVE HEALTHCARE GUIDELINES
- AVOID RISKY BEHAVIORS

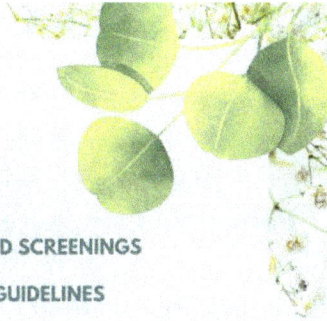

### The Importance of Exercise and Sleep

Regular exercise has numerous benefits for overall health and well-being. Here are some of the benefits:

- **Improved cardiovascular health:** Regular exercise can help strengthen the heart and improve blood flow, decreasing the risk of heart disease, stroke, and high blood pressure.
  - **Weight management:** Exercise can help burn calories and maintain a healthy weight, essential for reducing the risk of a range of chronic conditions.
- **Reduced risk of chronic disease:** Regular exercise is associated with a decreased risk of chronic diseases such as diabetes, cancer, and osteoporosis.
- **Improved mental health:** Exercise is effective in reducing symptoms of anxiety and depression, as well as improving overall mood and well-being.
- **Increased energy and stamina:** Regular exercise can improve muscle strength and endurance, increasing energy levels and life.
- **Better sleep quality:** Exercise can improve sleep quality and duration, which can positively impact overall health and well-being.
- **Stronger bones and muscles:** Exercise can help maintain bone density and muscle mass, which is especially important as we age.

Regular exercise is an essential component of a healthy lifestyle and can significantly impact a person's physical health and vitality. Physical vitality refers to having energy, strength, and stamina to perform daily tasks and engage in physical activities. It encompasses a sense of aliveness and feeling healthy and capable in one's body. Your physical weight does not accurately indicate health and vitality, but exercising regularly is crucial to your health and life.

## Sleep is essential for good health and contentment.

It is a necessary component of the body's natural healing and repair process and vital to maintaining physical and mental health. Here are some of the critical reasons why sleep is important:

- **Physical health:** Sleep helps the body to repair and rejuvenate. Studies show links between good sleep and a range of physical benefits such as improved immunity, better regulation of appetite and hormones, improved heart health, and reduced risk of diabetes and obesity.
- **Mental health:** Sleep is crucial in regulating mood and emotions and is essential for cognitive functioning, such as memory, attention, and decision-making. Sleep problems are linked to various mental health disorders, including depression, anxiety, and substance abuse.
- **Energy and productivity:** Good quality sleep is essential for the body to restore energy levels and maintain productivity. Getting sufficient rest can help individuals feel more alert, focused, and motivated throughout the day.
- **Safety:** Sleep deprivation can impair judgment, reaction time, and other critical cognitive functions, increasing the risk of accidents and injuries. Getting adequate sleep is essential for ensuring safety in daily life.

Quality and restful sleep is a cornerstone of good health and contentment. Individuals need to prioritize getting enough restful and restorative sleep each night. If you are having trouble sleeping, there are things you can do to help get your sleep habits back in check. One of those things is physical exercise.

## Proper Nutrition and Its Effects on the Body

Proper nutrition is essential for maintaining good health and preventing chronic diseases. A well-balanced diet that includes a variety of nutrient-dense foods can provide the body with the vitamins, minerals, and other nutrients it needs to function optimally. Here are some of the critical effects that proper nutrition can have on the body:

- **Improved energy levels:** Eating a balanced diet can give the body the energy needed to perform daily activities.
- **Improved mental health:** A balanced diet can help support brain function and improve mood.
  - **Reduced risk of chronic diseases:** A healthy diet high in fruits, vegetables, whole grains, lean proteins, and healthy fats can help reduce the risk of chronic diseases such as heart disease, type 2 diabetes, and certain types of cancer.
- **Healthy weight management:** Follow a balanced and nutritious diet and avoid fad diets that restrict your nutritional intake and may not be sustainable in the long run.
- **More robust immune system:** Consuming a diet rich in nutrients can help support the immune system and reduce the risk of infections and illnesses.

Proper nutrition is a critical component of good health and disease prevention. Individuals should prioritize consuming a diet rich in whole, nutrient-dense foods. We recommend finding a Holistic Nutritionist or someone who is trained in holistic nutrition. Co-author Sharry is one of them! Therefore, we are including a section on some great recipes that Sharry created that are both holistic and very yummy.

## The Ins and Outs of Digestion

We eat and drink every day, several times a day, out of necessity, and often without thinking. Our bodies require fuel to live from what we eat and drink.

Food entering into and exiting from the body is what we call digestion. Throughout our body, various stages of breakdown and absorption occur as our body takes the nutrients from the food, puts them where they are needed, and discards the remainder.

Digestion begins with a thought. Think of your favorite food, how it looks, smells, and tastes and your mouth will start to water. This water in your mouth is saliva. Saliva is the first fluid that our body uses to digest food. Saliva softens the food and breaks the food into smaller, softer pieces swallow and ingest.

In the stomach is a digestive fluid called hydrochloric acid. This acid breaks down the proteins in our food so the body can distribute them where needed. Hydrochloric acid can be pretty dangerous outside the body; fortunately, our stomach lining can withstand this caustic juice.

From the stomach, food continues into the "digestive tract," a long tube that squeezes food through the intestines and allows the absorption of nutrients along the way.

At the end of this digestive tract is the rectum, a pouch that holds all the unused and undigested elements from food, and when this pouch is full, it evacuates the fecal matter, or stool, from the body.

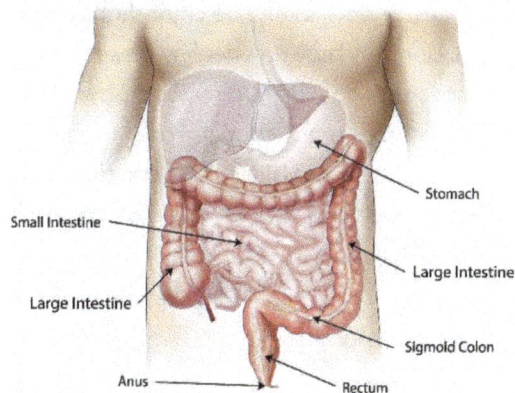

When "all systems are go," food enters and exits the body smoothly and rhythmically. However, this system can get out of balance, and troubles can arise. Heartburn, burping, bloating, constipation, and diarrhea are indicators that this system is out of balance. These symptoms can be from food sensitivities, illnesses, bacteria, viruses or molds, trauma, and some medications.

When these symptoms occur, look first at your diet. These symptoms can often be relieved by simply stopping consumption of the foods that cause the symptoms.

Urine should be clear and slightly yellow. Dark-colored or cloudy urine indicates dehydration and can quickly be cleared up by drinking more water. However, some supplements and medications can cause darker yellow urine. Research any drugs or supplements you are taking to see if they may cause darker-colored urine. Most people tend to be dehydrated, but on occasion, some over-hydrate. If your urine is clear and you have been drinking lots of water, you could be drinking too much. Finding the right amount for your body is the key.

Feces, or stool, should be cigar-shaped and moderately brown. A healthy bowel movement has very little odor. Be aware that some foods can change the color of the stool. Blackberries and blueberries can darken the stool, beets and strawberries may cause a reddish hue.

*Take a Moment*

It is healthy to have two to three bowel movements per day. It is also beneficial to urinate several times per day. Trying to "keep it in" for long periods can damage the bowels and bladder, as this puts excess stress on those organs trying to keep you from building up toxic waste and becoming ill. While sometimes we need to wait a few minutes before visiting the bathroom, we should go as soon as possible to keep a regular flow of release.

Let's do a self-check. How is your sleep? How can you improve it? How about your digestion? Anything you want to focus on?

_____
_____
_____
_____
_____
_____
_____
_____
_____
_____
_____
_____

# Sharry's Holistic Recipes

## *Apple and Green Tomato Chutney*

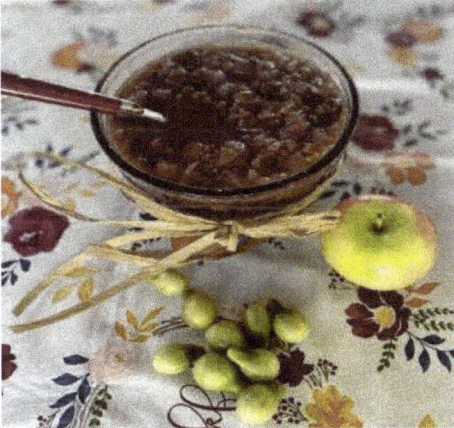
Image by Sharry Smith

2 cups peeled, diced apples
½ cup sugar
½ cup diced green tomatoes
2 tsp nutmeg
1 cup diced yellow squash
½ cup dried cranberries

Combine all ingredients in a saucepan. Cover with water. Cook on medium/low heat until vegetables are soft, stirring frequently and adding more water as necessary. As the chutney thickens, lower the cooking temperature.

Allow to cool. Keep the chutney in a glass container in the fridge. It will last for about a month. This chutney is excellent as a dip with pita chips, a spread on breads, or a garnish.

Cooking tip: When adding more water, add boiling water to not retard the cooking temperature.

Chutney, a dish originating in India, consists of various fruits and vegetables, spices, and sugar. Chutney is a condiment that can be used as a topping to meats and fish, spooned over crackers or bread, or served alone as a side dish. This delightful dish has found its way to the Caribbean islands, where tropical fruits such as mango and papaya are commonly used. This dish is known as relish in America, and vegetables such as tomatoes and corn are some favored ingredients. Adding a touch of chutney brings out an extra layer of flavor to foods, enhancing the enjoyment of a meal. And it is a great way to use local produce.

When our local produce is ripe in the summer, we can make some delicious chutneys with foods from our gardens or the local farmers' markets. As the summer turns to autumn and we want to find ways to use the last crops, chutney can be canned, bottled, and stored for winter use. Bringing out a bottle of homemade chutney will perk up the Thanksgiving table or the family Christmas dinner. And when a last-minute gift is needed, a bottle of homemade chutney is a great idea.

Whether making chutney or relish, using locally grown produce brings a sense of community and belonging. A chutney dish on the table or a bottle of chutney wrapped and given as a loving gift can be a delightful addition to that sense of belonging.

A homemade dish from local harvest, family around the table, gifts to friends and neighbors, now that's love.

## Lavender Spearmint Tea

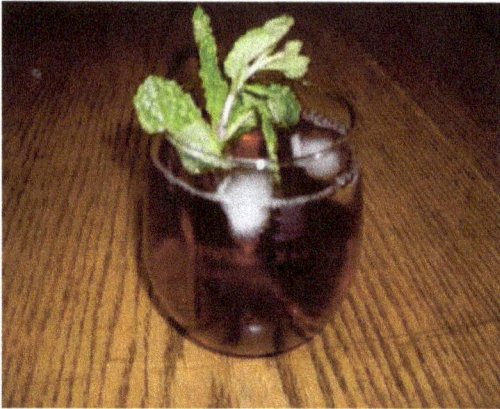
Image by Sharry Smith

1 quart water
1/3 cup agave syrup
3 Tbsp. dried lavender
3 Tbsp. dried spearmint

Put dried lavender and spearmint into a mesh strainer or bit of cheesecloth. Stir in agave syrup. Heat water and herbs in a saucepan until steam begins. Do not boil.

Allow tea to cool; remove herbs. Serve hot or cold.

Light and refreshing, this herbal tea can be made from herbs in your garden or the local farmer's market.

At the end of a long day or during times of stress, lavender can help relieve headaches and anxieties. Adding a touch of spearmint increases this relief and relieves symptoms of nausea, indigestion, gas, and sore throats.

These unpleasant symptoms result from a hectic daily lifestyle in our modern culture. Work deadlines, traffic, worrisome news stories, family troubles — all of these situations may cause us to feel as if we have to hurry and solve the issues or live up to someone else's expectations. When this happens, our central nervous system goes into overtime and takes all the energy from our body, leaving our digestion with little energy to draw on. Using these calming herbs in a relaxing tea will soothe the anxiety and return energy to our digestion, removing the nausea, headaches, and other symptoms we may be experiencing.

Find yourself a quiet little space where you can be alone for a little while. Make yourself some of this tea, put your feet up, sip the tea slowly, and enjoy the pleasant aroma of your cup or glass.

Drink the tea chilled on a hot day or warmed on a cold evening. Breathe deeply and slowly, letting each sip travel slowly down your throat and caress all the tissues, coating your digestive tract in a loving and healing liquid that digests quickly and brings you back to yourself.

Life is meant to be enjoyed. Troubles may arise occasionally, and when they do, this little tea will help you through. Cheers!

## Chunky Mixed Greens Caprese Salad

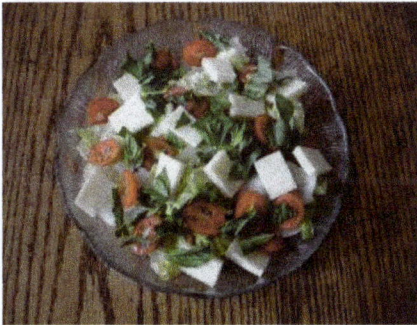
Image by Sharry Smith

2 cups mixed greens or salad mix
2 oz. mozzarella cheese sliced thin and cut in thirds
8 grape tomatoes, halved
A few sprigs fresh basil, chopped

Fill a shallow bowl with 2 cups of mixed greens. Arrange mozzarella slices and tomato halves on top of greens. Scatter the chopped basil over the salad. Drizzle with olive oil.

A light and easy salad for a hot summer day.

We often look for something cool and refreshing for lunch or dinner on a hot summer day. Salads fit the bill perfectly. Try fresh greens and other veggies, a little protein, and voilà, a scrumptious dish that's nutritious, light, and easy on the tummy.

Green leafy vegetables like lettuce, kale, chard, and spinach contain tons of minerals we lose when we sweat. Our body uses minerals to conduct its electrical signals. These electrical signals are how our body communicates from the skin to the brain and back. Our brain checks the balance of minerals in different parts of our body and determines if we need more in that area, and if so, sends the required minerals and puts them to work. Minerals such as calcium, potassium, boron, magnesium, and a host of others are crucial in maintaining the balance of blood and other fluids. We need a proportion of all these minerals to stay healthy and operate at peak performance.

Raw vegetables are tasty and the crunch helps keep our teeth and jaws strong. Raw vegetables also contain maximum amounts of fiber. Fiber helps to keep our digestive tract clear of excess debris and assists in elimination. In the olden days, fiber was known as roughage. So, roughly stated, fiber helps us poop.

Adding some protein to a salad makes it a complete meal. Proteins like chicken, turkey, tuna, beans, seeds, nuts, and cheese in moderation also add flavor to the salad. (Did you know that soft white cheeses also contain probiotics?) Toss in some cut-up fruit for some added sweetness. There are thousands of combinations of veggies and protein to make a salad. The sky is the limit. So get in the kitchen and see what you can produce in your salad. Mix and match, grate and create, all to your liking. Salad is my favorite meal.

## Tomato Vegetable Soup with Meatballs

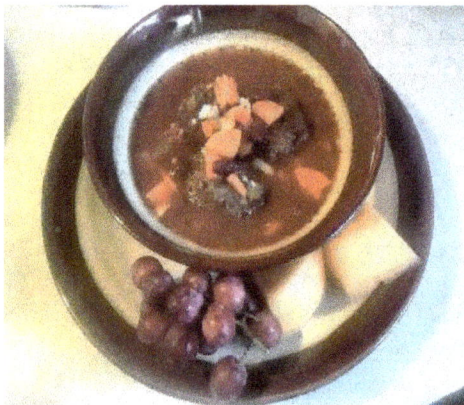
Image by Sharry Smith

6 cups broth
1 lb. ground bison
3 medium carrots, diced
2 eggs, beaten
2 stalks celery, diced
2 cups crushed rice cereal
2 cups diced tomatoes
1 Tbsp. salt
1 15-oz can beans
1 tsp black pepper
8 cloves garlic, chopped
4 Tbsp. olive oil

In a large stockpot, cook all the vegetables and spices on medium heat until the vegetables are soft. Add a tiny bit of olive oil if desired.

While the broth and vegetables are cooking, place the ground bison in a medium mixing bowl. Add the eggs, rice cereal, and spices. Mix well, and form into meatballs. (To make the meatballs uniform in size, use a melon baller or ice cream scoop.)

Heat a large skillet and add enough olive oil to coat the pan. Brown the meatballs on all sides until the juices run clear.

Place three meatballs in a serving bowl and ladle soup over the meatballs. Serve with a side of fruit for a hearty and healthy meal.

"Soup is good food" was a campaign slogan many years ago for a famous brand of canned soups. They were right. The many combinations of vegetables, herbs, spices, and proteins created a delightful and comfortable dish that is healthy and healing. The best way to enjoy this healing and cozy dish is to make it yourself, at home, with fresh ingredients. Canned soups contain preservatives that are necessary for sustaining shelf life but are harmful to the human body over time. Homemade soups have none of that, just whole fresh foods.

The broth is the base for the soup. That warm, yummy liquid that all the veggies are swimming in is packed full of easily digested nutrition, especially for a troubled tummy or someone ill. Remember when you were sick as a child and your mom brought you chicken soup? It was soothing and healing, almost like your tummy being hugged better.

Broth is made from simmering the bones of chicken, turkey, or beef. Slow simmering over a long period, a few hours, brings out the nutrition from the bones. Collagen, minerals, and vitamins leach into the liquid and can be easily taken into the digestive tract. These nutrients help to build new cells to replace the sick ones. This is how the body heals.

Soup is also a low-calorie dish and can help reduce excess fat and pounds that tend to creep up on us.

Vegans and vegetarians will be delighted to enjoy a vegetable broth made from simmering veggie stalks. I often use the core of a head of cauliflower, the stalks from broccoli and celery, and even asparagus stalks in my veggie broth. Add a little sea salt and a couple of bay leaves while the broth is simmering to enhance flavor.

Once the broth is finished, you can add anything you want to your soup. There are endless possibilities and options. Veggies, beans, meats, herbs and spices, and even some pasta, rice, or other grains can be incorporated into your homemade soup. That's one of the best things about cooking at home; you can mix and match your ingredients to your taste and liking.

Add some milk (dairy or plant-based) for creamed soups to the broth and put it in a blender, or use a submersible blender in the pan. Then, toss in some pre-cooked veggies and other ingredients. This is a slight difference from soup, because if the veggies are raw, the cream will separate and lose its form. If you already cooked the veggies with the broth you are in great shape.

Sometimes, we can drink a cup of warm broth. Drinking warm broth is a great way to get some nutrition if we're not feeling up to par or in a hurry. Broth can also be used in place of water when cooking rice or pasta for flavor and nutrition.

Find yourself some soup recipes and try them out. Once you get the hang of making the broth, soup becomes relatively easy. Making a big pot of soup will stay in the refrigerator for a few days and can be frozen for later. It's a good idea to have some soup in the freezer when a day pops up that you or someone in your home is not feeling well or if company drops in at the last minute.

Soup is a great way to use small bits of leftover veggies and scraps of meat. It is said that Americans throw away tons of food each year, so by making soup out of our leftovers, we can reduce some of the waste. And some of the waist. Enjoy your soup.

## Corn and Bean Nachos

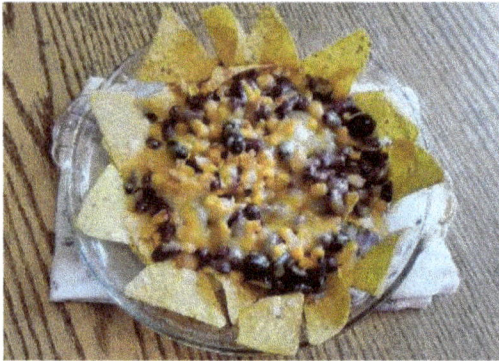

Image by Sharry Smith

Large can of kidney or black beans
Small can corn
18 black olives, halved
$\frac{1}{4}$ cup diced onion
4 oz. taco sauce
6 oz. shredded cheese
Corn chips

Combine beans, corn, olives, onion, and taco sauce in a medium bowl. Layer corn chips into a glass baking dish. Top with bean and veggie mix.

Bake in the oven at 350° for about 20 minutes. Sprinkle cheese over the top, return to oven, and heat until melted.

Homemade nachos are another great snack we can prepare using healthy vegetables, beans, and salsa. It is a simple, tasty, fun food for a quick snack or light dinner. This dish will also travel to potlucks and get-togethers - a pleasurable dish for any occasion.

## Snack Foods

Sometimes, we want something to eat, but only a partial meal. Or, we may need something we can serve at a party or bring to a potluck or get-together. We need finger foods that don't require silverware and a lot of fuss. It's just something that everyone can enjoy while socializing. These foods are called snack foods and come in various tastes and textures.

40

There are sweet snacks like cookies and ice cream treats. There are salty snacks like chips and nuts. A healthier version of snacks would be raw vegetables or cut-up fruits. Some bites of cheese or meat could be a snack. Whatever we choose, a snack can be eaten with our hands when we feel a little hungry or want to munch on something while socializing.

Packaged snacks in grocery stores are convenient for snacking when on the go. Packaged snacks are inexpensive and tempting but may also be full of sugar, harmful fats, and salt. These packaged snacks may be okay occasionally when we find ourselves in a pinch for something quick, but try to find healthier options. One way to ensure we get healthy snacks if we are on the go is to carry small bags of nuts or plain popcorn. These do not need refrigeration and travel well. If we have access to a refrigerator at work, or if we can keep a cooler in our car, veggie sticks, string cheese, boiled eggs, or bits of cooked chicken would be something to consider.

Some snacks can be made at home, such as homemade French fries baked in the oven. Just wash and slice a potato, bake it on a cookie sheet, sprinkle on a little sea salt, and enjoy the fast-food taste without the heavy oils and food additives.

If you want a sweet snack, homemade is still the best option. Bake your cookies using healthier ingredients like honey or stevia instead of sugar. Substitute carob chips for chocolate chips. Try almond or coconut flour to replace the wheat flour containing gluten.

Snacks are okay, but avoid the excess sugars, salts, preservatives, and food additives in packaged snacks. The internet is full of healthy snack ideas, and a little time surfing the web will give you some great ideas.

Preparing healthy snacks at home takes a little time, but far less than you would spend in the doctor's office from overeating junk. Just sayin.'

## Eat the Rainbow Platter

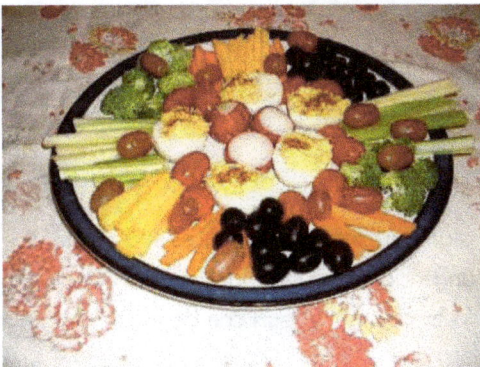

Carrots
Celery
Olives
Cherry tomatoes
Broccoli
Radishes
Deviled eggs

Image by Sharry Smith

You may have heard the expression "Eat the rainbow," referring to various colors in our chosen foods. Foods come in different colors depending on what nutrients they contain. Green foods have phytonutrients, nutrients that the plant creates from sunlight that help repair and rebuild damaged cells and tissues and aid in digestion. Red and orange foods contain resveratrol, an anti-inflammatory antioxidant that helps the body eliminate old or damaged cells and helps protect the heart and blood from cellular damage. Olives are a great source of healthy omega fatty acids that keep our vessels and brain pliable for fluid flow. Cheese and eggs are a great source of protein, necessary for building strength in the body.

In this vegetable platter, you will find various colors, textures, and essential nutrients vital for a healthy diet. You can add or substitute different vegetables, fruits, or proteins when you make one. For example, some cooked diced chicken, smoked salmon, pickles, and other finger foods can make tasty options. Make a vegetable plate that suits your taste and body's needs. Get creative and make eating healthy fun.

## Fruit and Yogurt Salad

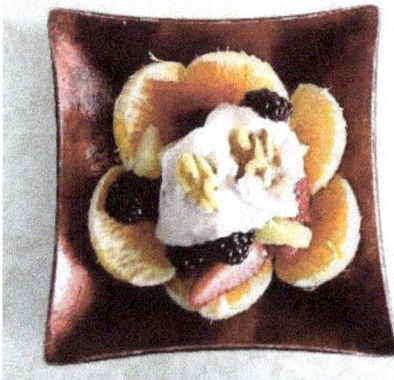

Image by Sharry Smith

1 medium orange
1/3 cup pineapple bits
3 large strawberries
1/2 cup strawberry yogurt
6 to 8 blackberries
1/4 cup walnut pieces

First, peel and separate the orange. On a small plate, arrange orange slices in a circle. Slice the strawberries and place them in the middle of the orange slices and the blackberries. Spoon the yogurt onto the fruit top with pineapple bits and walnuts. Coconut yogurt can be used for a vegan variation.

This is a perfect desert for a healthy diet or can serve as a light breakfast or lunch.

Many folks are dealing with digestive issues due to poor diet, food sensitivities, medications, toxic exposures, illness, etc. These digestive troubles can often be helped, relieved, and potentially cured with probiotics in the regular diet.

Around 70% of our immune system is in our digestive tract. When food, drink, or other substances enter our stomach, this immune system is there to ward off unwanted or unrecognized elements and prevent us from becoming ill. If this system is off balance, health troubles can arise. Stomach disorders, headaches and body aches, skin rashes, and mood disorders can sometimes result from an immune system not working at its full potential.

In our digestive tract is candida yeast, which is part of the immune balance. When we are exposed to trauma or illness, this yeast gets overgrown and begins to swell. This swelling is inflammation and does not have to be seen to be felt. Generally, a large swollen abdomen indicates abdominal inflammation, but a thin person can also have inflammation.

Eating probiotic foods will help to restore and maintain the balance of good bacteria and candida yeast. Fermented foods such as yogurt, sour cream, buttermilk, and kefir are some dairy forms of probiotics — the fermenting process creates good bacteria. Yogurts made from coconut milk or almond milk are also good probiotic sources for folks sensitive to dairy products. Sauerkraut, kimchee, kombucha, and even pickles are probiotic and suitable for vegan diets. You may also look into probiotic supplements to help you get your digestive tract back into balance.

However you choose to add probiotics to your diet, your body will thank you for feeling better, looser, and lighter. This is just one of the many ways we can improve our health, and it only takes a little money, awareness, and determination. Be aware of what you eat; it dramatically affects your health. And you are worth it.

## *Zucchini Pizza Bites*

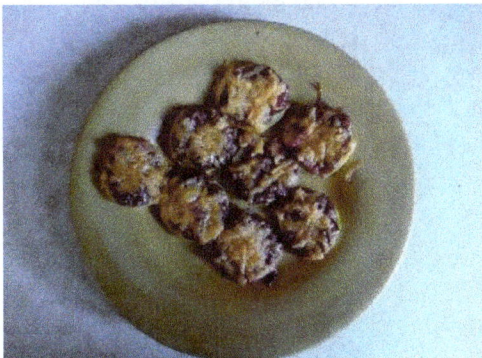

Image by Sharry Smith

Zucchini slices
Marinara sauce
Shredded cheese
Basil
Oregano

Arrange zucchini slices on a sheet pan or cookie sheet. Top with marinara sauce, cheese, basil, and oregano to taste.

Bake at 375° for 20 minutes or until cheese is melted and bubbly.
Allow to cool slightly, then enjoy.

When you've just got to have pizza…and nothing else will do! Here's a fun twist that makes it healthier and as tasty as the real deal. This makes perfect little pizza bites that satisfy the craving without putting on the extra pounds. It's excellent for gluten-sensitive and reduced carb diets as well. Delicious pizza tastes are also a perfect snack for entertaining.

If the kiddos turn their noses up at the thought of zucchini, don't tell them. Just say, "Here, I made you some baby pizzas." They might go for it, and you can sneak vegetables into them. As they get older, you can disclose what is in the pizza bites, and possibly, they will be more accepting of the vegetables by then.

A funny story: My mother often made corned beef hash from scratch as a child. I loved it. One day, I heard about someone eating beef tongue, and I was horrified at the thought of eating something from a cow's mouth. My mother laughed and said, "You've been eating it all your life." "WHAT! WHEN?" I exclaimed. "I use it in the corned beef hash." She laughed again, and after I got over my shock, I figured it might not be so bad if I didn't have to see the tongue. I still ate her corned beef hash but with a new awareness.

It's funny what people will eat without knowing what's in it.

## Gluten Free Meatloaf

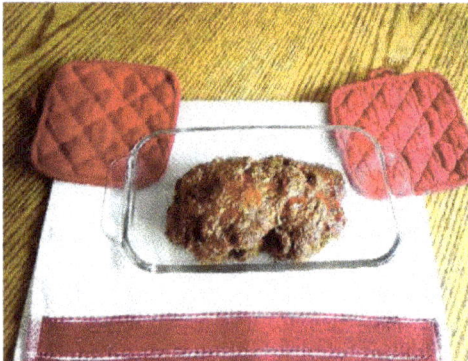
Image by Sharry Smith

1 lb. ground bison
1 ½ cups ground rice cereal
1 tsp salt
¼ tsp black pepper
2 cloves chopped garlic
2 eggs
1 tsp parsley
½ tsp sage
½ tsp thyme
Catsup

Mix all ingredients in a medium mixing bowl, using your clean-washed hands to squeeze it together. Shape into a rectangular loaf shape.

Place the meatloaf into a loaf pan or other baking pan.

Bake at 350° for 45 minutes. Spread catsup over meatloaf using a brush, then return to the oven for another 5 minutes.

Remove from oven and let sit for about 10 minutes. Slice and serve.

Meatloaf has been a favored comfort food for generations. It is relatively inexpensive, filling, and often found on family tables. Traditionally, meatloaf is made from ground beef, but ground turkey, chicken or other meats can also be used. There are also meat-free options using plant-based foods such as soy or black beans.

When making meatloaf, whatever the ingredients, you need something to hold it together and give it bulk. Bread crumbs have long been used to provide bulk and help to give the feeling of being "full" after eating it. Some folks have sensitivities to bread crumbs made from wheat, so we need to find another choice.

I am one of those who deal with wheat sensitivities, and I enjoy an occasional meatloaf. After much trial and error, I have discovered that dry rice cereal fills the bill. I use a grocery store brand, but you can choose whatever brand of dry rice cereal you desire. I crush the grain using a rolling pin and make "bread crumbs" from the rice cereal. It gives the same bulk in the dish and the same feeling after eating it.

I may mix in some small broccoli florets, diced carrots or celery, and chopped spinach leaves or other greens for extra nutrition.

## Irish Chicken

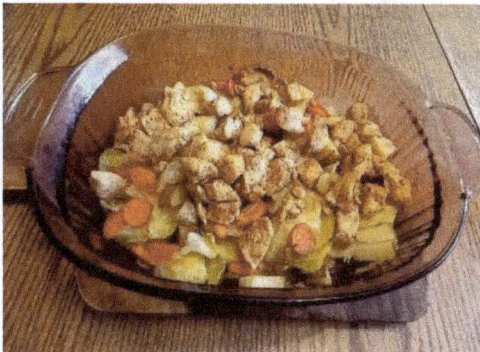

Image by Sharry Smith

2 pieces boneless skinless chicken breast
2 cups chopped cabbage
2 medium diced potatoes
2 medium diced carrots
1 cup diced onion
¼ cup olive oil
1 dash salt
1 tsp black pepper
2 tsp garlic powder
2 tsp thyme
1 tsp paprika

Chop the chicken into bite-size pieces. Brown the chicken with the spices in half of the olive oil in a large skillet. Set aside.

Into the skillet, put the cabbage, potatoes, carrots, and onion with the other half of the olive oil and cook until soft.

Replace the chicken in the skillet with the vegetables. Cook for another 2 to 3 minutes, stirring frequently.

Serve with a side salad or fruit. Serves 2 to 3 people.

## Cultural Cuisine

Since the dawn of time, humankind has enjoyed sharing meals with others. Whether it be family, friends, or neighbors, a group of people sitting down to eat together is something we look forward to. Birthdays, holidays, and other festive occasions are times when we can experience this. In our daily lives, the family having dinner together is a time to share the meal, share our everyday experiences, and learn about each other. The family dinner can unite and bring it closer as a loving unit.

Family recipes are handed down through generations, and depending on where the family roots are, these recipes are unique to that area. Africa, Europe, Asia, North and South America, and our island nations have dishes, spices, and cooking methods that reflect that area's culture. Cultural recipes speak of our ancestors and help to continue the lineage of the tribe or family.

In my family, my father's side was primarily Irish. I remember my paternal grandmother's boiled shrimp with potatoes and sauerkraut, the smell of the shrimp with all the spices filling the house with her loving touch. On my mother's side, there were some Africans, and some of the recipes came from the enslaved Africans in the south where she was from. My grandmother's stuffed bell peppers were filled with ground beef, rice, onion, corn, and tomatoes from an Ethiopian dish called *abish*.

Our culture is a source of connection to our past and our families through food, recipes, celebrations, clothing, and ways of speaking. Each culture has a long history of people and events that have created it, and each culture should be respected for what it is: simply a way of living for a particular people.

I enjoy experiencing different cultural foods. There are so many incredible tastes and textures, and each one, for me, brings a closer connection to my brothers and sisters with whom I share this planet.

Enjoy your culture, enjoy your cultural foods, and enjoy life. We're all in this together.

## Making Lifestyle Changes

When we begin changing our diet, others may be against us. Many have someone, whether it be family, friends, coworkers, or neighbors, who tend to disbelieve and discourage our changes. We go to dinner with someone, and our choice of food may be questioned. Or they might say something like, "I don't know what to feed you." or "You can't eat anything." Try not to pay much attention to this negativity. It comes from fear of change on their part.

It is human nature to be afraid of change. We live in our comfort zones, and anything that disrupts that comfort zone may cause fear. Be patient with those who feel and express this fear and negativity. Explain that you are making a change for yourself and that they don't have to change themselves. This change is for you. Be kind and gentle, tactful in your wording, and stick to your plan.

Making changes may be difficult, and there may be relapses. When that happens, acknowledge that you are imperfect and return to the wagon. One is perfect.

Life is a journey; the little ups and downs, setbacks, and mistakes are part of that journey. Enjoy your trip with all its oopsies, and know that you will succeed by focusing on your goal. It will take time and your new habits will eventually become your natural lifestyle.

## Healthy Hygiene Habits

Good hygiene habits are essential for maintaining good health and preventing the spread of illness and infection. Here are some healthy hygiene habits that individuals can practice:

- Regularly washing hands with soap and water for at least 20 seconds – can help prevent the spread of germs and bacteria.
- Brushing teeth twice daily and flossing once daily can help prevent tooth decay, gum disease, and other oral health problems.
- Regular bathing or showering can help remove dirt, sweat, and bacteria from the body.
- Covering the mouth and nose with a tissue or elbow when coughing or sneezing can help prevent the spread of germs to others.
- Keeping nails clean and trimmed can help prevent the accumulation of dirt and bacteria.
- Wearing personal protective equipment, such as gloves and masks, when necessary can help prevent the spread of illness and infection.

Practicing good hygiene habits is vital to maintaining good health and preventing the spread of illness and infection. In that case, it is not only healthy for you, but for others around you too! We have learned much about the importance of not spreading illness in recent years and during COVID's peak.

## Preventing Chronic Disease

Physical health plays a significant role in preventing chronic diseases. Chronic diseases, such as heart disease, stroke, diabetes, and cancer, are among the leading causes of death and disability worldwide. Regular physical activity, proper nutrition, and healthy lifestyle habits can help prevent and manage chronic diseases. Here are some ways in which physical health can help prevent chronic diseases:

- Regular physical activity, such as brisk walking, cycling, or swimming, can help improve cardiovascular health, maintain a healthy weight, reduce blood pressure, and lower the risk of chronic diseases such as heart disease and stroke.
- Eating a well-balanced diet rich in fruits, vegetables, whole grains, lean proteins, and healthy fats can help reduce the risk of many chronic diseases including Type 2 diabetes and certain types of cancer.
- Maintaining a healthy weight through regular physical activity and proper nutrition can help reduce the risk of chronic diseases such as heart disease, Type 2 diabetes, and certain types of cancer.
- Avoiding risky behaviors such as smoking, excessive alcohol consumption, and drug use can help prevent various health problems, including chronic diseases.

Maintaining good physical health is essential for preventing chronic diseases and reducing the risk of severe health problems. Seriously, don't forget about your physical health! It is genuinely vital to preventing chronic diseases.

## The Importance of Check-ups

Regular screenings and check-ups are essential for maintaining good physical health. These appointments can help identify potential health problems early on before they become more serious.

Screenings and check-ups can also help keep track of important health metrics, such as blood pressure, cholesterol levels, and blood sugar levels. Here are some additional reasons why regular screenings and check-ups are essential:

- Screenings and check-ups can help prevent and detect health problems early on, improving treatment outcomes and increasing the chances of a full recovery.
- Managing chronic conditions with regular check-ups can help individuals with chronic conditions such as diabetes, high blood pressure, and heart disease keep their needs under control and manage them effectively.
- Regular check-ups can help healthcare providers monitor an individual's overall health status and identify any changes that could indicate the onset of a health problem.

Regular screenings and check-ups are essential for maintaining good physical health and preventing serious health problems. Individuals should work with their holistic professionals to develop a screening and check-up schedule that meets their needs and helps them stay healthy.

Be aware that some holistic professionals don't do regular bloodwork or tests, and others do. Research all professionals before you schedule with them — learn what they offer and check reviews.

## The Physical and Mental Health Connection

There is a strong connection between physical health and mental health. Physical fitness can significantly impact mental health and vice versa. For example, chronic physical health conditions such as heart disease, stroke, and cancer can increase the risk of depression and anxiety. Additionally, poor physical health behaviors, such as a lack of exercise, poor nutrition, and substance abuse, can contribute to poor mental health outcomes.

On the other hand, good physical health practices such as regular exercise, proper nutrition, and adequate sleep can help improve mental health outcomes. Engaging in physical activity releases endorphins, which can help improve mood and reduce stress. Eating a healthy diet can help improve brain function and reduce the risk of mental health disorders.

Taking care of both physical and mental health is essential to achieve optimal overall health and well-being. Individuals should work with their healthcare providers to develop a plan that meets their needs and helps them maintain good physical and mental health.

## The Benefits of Physical Activity

Physical activity has numerous benefits for mental health. Here are some of the key benefits:

- Exercise has been shown to decrease symptoms of depression and anxiety by releasing endorphins, which are feel-good hormones that can help improve mood and reduce stress.
- Exercise has been shown to enhance cognitive function, including improving memory, attention, and processing speed, which can help reduce the risk of cognitive decline.
- Exercise can help improve self-esteem and body image, leading to better emotional well-being and increased confidence.
- Exercise can be a great way to reduce stress and tension, which can help improve mental health and overall well-being.
- Regular physical activity can enhance the quality of sleep, which is essential for overall mental health and well-being.

Regular physical activity can significantly benefit mental health and reduce symptoms of depression and anxiety, improve cognitive function, boost self-esteem, reduce stress, and improve sleep quality. Working with a holistic practitioner will help you develop a plan that meets your needs and helps you maintain good physical and mental health.

## Holistic Practices to Build Immunity by Stephanie

Holistic Health is based on the law of nature that a whole is made up of interdependent parts. The earth is made up of systems, such as air, land, water, plants, and animals. If life is to be sustained, they cannot be separated, for what is happening to one is also felt by the other systems. In the same way, an individual is a whole made up of interdependent parts, which are the physical, mental, emotional, social, and spiritual. When one part is not working at its best, it impacts all of the other parts of that person. For example, when an individual fears the potential of getting sick or being out of work, their nervousness may result in a physical reaction - such as a headache or a stomach ache. When people deal with overwhelming stress, the body, mind, and emotions may be affected negatively.

When we are imbalanced within our mind, emotions, and spirit, our physical body will automatically be affected. The immune system's performance drops when we feel heavy emotions such as anxiety, worry, fear, grief, or anger. This drop in the immune system also leads to the person experiencing depression, which adds to the further declining health of the individual's immune system. When we are off balance in our minds, emotions, and spirit, our immune system becomes compromised, and we are more prone to illness.

The best thing that we can do to boost our immune system is to bring positivity to our mental, emotional, and spiritual outlooks. This can be done with daily yoga, meditation, affirmations, or prayer. You only need to start for 20-30 minutes of practice daily. With these practices, you will focus on moving your body, letting stress go, bringing movement to the immune system, and changing mental, emotional, and spiritual outlooks to a more positive note.

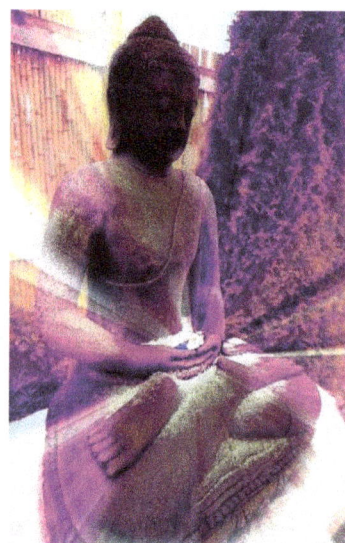

Image by Wonderlane

## Spiritual Morning Routine Template

Follow this template for step-by-step instructions to create your 20-30-minute daily practice.

**When are you going to practice?**

*Example:* "I am going to practice after breakfast daily."

**Where are you going to practice?**

*Example:* "I will practice using a yoga mat in my bedroom and will have a lit candle on my desk."

- Make sure your phone is on "do not disturb."
- Open up your "Insight Timer," or other meditation app for meditation practice.
- Ensure others in the household know not to disturb you during this time.

## YOGA: 10-15 MINUTES

Example: Downward Dog, Child's Pose, Pigeon Pose, Happy Baby. End in Shavasana.

Complete List of Yoga Poses (Workout Trends website: https://workouttrends.com/yoga-poses)

10 Minute Morning for Beginners (SarahBeth Yoga YouTube channel: https://www.youtube.com/watch?v=VaoV1PrYft4)

10 Minute Yoga for Neck, Shoulders, Upper Back (SarahBeth Yoga YouTube channel: https://www.youtube.com/watch?v=VaoV1PrYft4)

## MEDITATION: 7-10 minutes

Headspace Meditation Tips (Headspace YouTube channel: https://www.youtube.com/watch?v=pDm_na_Blq8)

Headspace Letting Go Headspace YouTube channel: https://www.youtube.com/watch?v=wyj8l9miy4w)

## AFFIRMATIONS AND MANIFESTING: 5 minutes.

Manifestation & Affirmations ("People Who Practice These 3 Daily Habits Are the Happiest By Far" YourTango website: https://www.yourtango.com/self/people-practice-daily-habits-happiest-by-far)

What is Manifestation? ("What Is "Manifestation" and Why Should I Care?" Kelsey Aida website: https://www.kelseyaida.com/theinspirationalblog/what-is-manifestation)

30 Powerful Affirmations ("Make positive affirmations part of your mental strength workout" Betterup website: https://www.betterup.com/blog/positive-affirmations)

**State three things you are feeling grateful for today.** (This will differ daily.)
Example: "I am grateful for the restful sleep I received last night."
State ten affirmations aloud.
Examples: "I am loved," "I trust the universe," "Money flows easily to me," "I love my life."
**State three things you are asking for daily.**
Example: "Today, I am asking for extra energy because I have many things on my to-do list." "Today, I am asking to receive some financial abundance."
**State prayers or requests for others.**
Example: "Today, I am asking that my sister be given some extra joy because she had a hard day yesterday." "Today, I am asking that my friend be given some extra confidence as she has a job interview today."
**Take three deep breaths.**

That's all! I hope this helps set up your daily routine of spiritual practice. Remember to have your way written somewhere (other than your phone) to refer to when practicing.

There are specific bodywork modalities of practice to improve the immune system. At Holistic Bodyworks, as with any holistic health practice, we can help you determine which type of bodywork and energy work is best for you and how often you should get work done. We also have nutrition and holistic health coaches that can help you set up a plan of action for your improved health.

What you eat is also a great place to start to boost your immune system. Eating a well-balanced diet full of fresh vegetables, fruits, and grass-fed and hormone-free meats will make a massive difference in your mental, emotional, and physical outlooks and can affect the health of our whole self. Researching to find a good balanced diet as a foundation for your health is a great idea.

## Holistic Nutrition

Eating for the mind, body, and soul in today's fast-paced, high-demand world, we have become a culture focused on convenience, including how we eat.

When hunger strikes, opening a can, unwrapping a package, or popping a lid is much easier than preparing a fresh meal. However, according to holistic nutritionists, the cost of convenience is not so much the impact on our pocketbook as it is the impact on our health. Holistic nutrition is all about eating healthy food as close to its natural state as possible for optimum health and well-being. Hallmarks of holistic nutrition include eating food that is unrefined, unprocessed, organic, and locally grown.

By following a holistic nutrition plan, you may experience many health benefits, including weight loss and weight management, disease prevention, increased energy levels, improved mood, better sleep, strengthened immune system, and improved digestion. Additionally, holistic nutritionists believe that many chronic illnesses can be prevented or improved through diet.

Some specific vitamins and supplements can help boost the immune system, which may already be in the foods you eat or can be taken in supplement form to be added to your diet.

To fuel your immune system, you want an ample supply of vitamin A, B complex, Vitamin C, Vitamin E, and Zinc.

You can also incorporate immune-strengthening herbs to boost your defenses further. You don't want to use these unless you have been exposed to someone with a cold, flu, or other virus. That's the time to tweak your immune system with several immune-boosting herbs, including Echinacea, goldenseal, chamomile, and ginger. Echinacea and goldenseal are the most potent immune enhancers and should be taken ONLY when you have been exposed to someone who is sick.

Chamomile and ginger can be taken more frequently for a healthy immune system.

Homeopathic remedies are a great option to take as another form of prevention for a viral sickness. Oscillococcinum is an excellent homeopathic remedy for boosting the immune system to help prevent the flu. Other homeopathic remedies can help fight a viral disease, but I wanted to provide the one that really helps boost the immune system and can be taken if you have been exposed to someone sick.

When we don't incorporate a regular spiritual practice, get regular bodywork/energy work, eat a holistic nutrition-based diet, and include immune-boosting vitamins and supplements, herbs, and homeopathic remedies, the immune system's effectiveness drops. If you do incorporate these holistic practices, you can build your immune system up so that if you are exposed to someone with a virus, you will have a better chance to fight off illness naturally.

Resources for learning about holistic nutrition

http://www.holistichelp.net/holistic-nutrition.html

http://www.holistic-wellness-basics.com/holistic-nutrition.html

## Integrating Physical Health Practices

Integrating physical health practices with other aspects of holistic health can lead to a more comprehensive approach to overall wellness. Holistic health emphasizes the interconnectedness of the body, mind, and spirit and incorporates various practices and therapies to support health and wellness.

Incorporating physical health practices such as regular exercise and proper nutrition with other approaches such as meditation, mindfulness, and spiritual practices can help support overall wellness.

These practices can help reduce stress, improve mood, enhance cognitive function, and improve physical health. For example, practicing yoga can be a way to integrate physical activity with mindfulness and spirituality. Yoga involves physical postures, movements, mindfulness, and meditation practices, which can help reduce stress and promote relaxation. Similarly, a healthy diet can be combined with other approaches, such as meditation or gratitude practices.

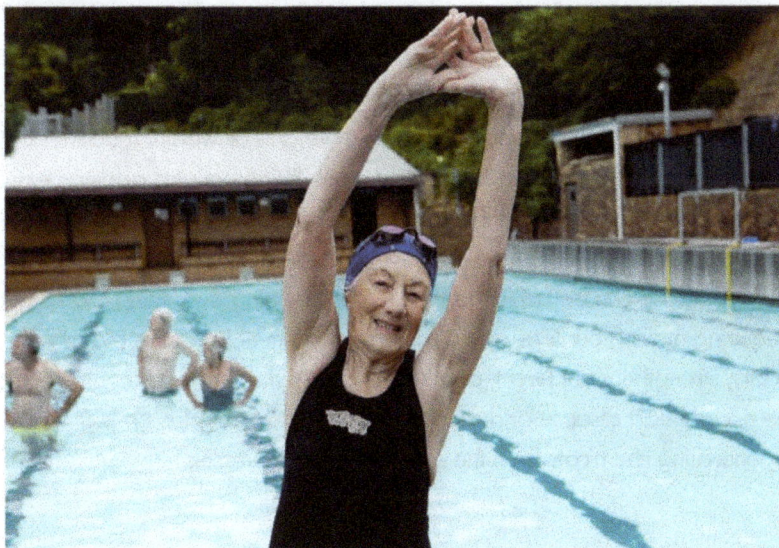

## Move It or Lose It by Sharry

Exercise is one of the most important things you can do for your health and life. Unfortunately, far too many people don't get enough exercise, or they don't exercise at all. This is sad as movement is free, can be done on your schedule, and can be lots of fun! Additional benefits like weight loss, increased strength and energy, and reduced pain only add to the package.

Our muscles and joints were designed to move and move frequently. If these muscles and joints are not moved regularly, they will stiffen and become less able to move. Think of a toy wagon left out in the yard. Over time, the wheels will rust and not want to move. Our tissues act in the same way. Without regular movement, the tissues will oxidize or rust and be less able to move. This results in pain and stiffness. So, using our muscles and joints regularly is like lubricating the joints or oiling the wheels on the wagon.

Moving the body lets the body release healing and regenerating chemicals into the bloodstream. Inside our blood vessels are cells that contain healing and restoring chemicals that are only activated by movement. Movement increases blood circulation and speeds it up, and by doing so, the blood sort of "takes the lid" off these cells, and then the healing chemicals can get out into the blood.

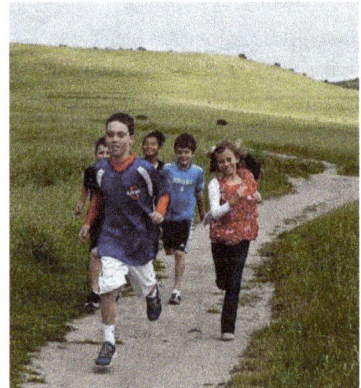

Image by blmcalifornia

Another benefit to exercise is the movement of lymph, our body's waste system. Lymph is a fluid that travels through its own set of vessels; its job is to carry toxins and discarded elements out of the body. Unlike our blood vessels that rely on the heart to pump blood through the body, lymph relies on movement to push it through to the blood stream. Exercise and moving the body enables this lymph to move toxins through the body for elimination.

Strengthening, weight-bearing, cardiovascular, and stretching exercises are all necessary for complete physical fitness.

Strengthening consists of lifting weights, such as free weights or weight machines at the gym. Even light hand weights will have a good effect. Standing while lifting weights adds an extra benefit because standing works the long muscles in our legs and increases bone density, increasing our overall strength and energy.

Cardiovascular exercise can be achieved by walking, jogging, swimming, dancing, tennis, or any other activity requiring moving our legs and arms. This movement increases blood flow, increases breathing capacity, strengthens our heart, and increases brain activity. This can be a massive benefit for reducing the risk of heart disease and dementia. This movement plays a big part in releasing the healing and regenerating chemicals from the cells in our blood vessels.

Stretching can come from simple, easy movements like yoga, tai chi, or Qi Gong. Stretching our body loosens the fibers and lets muscles and joints move and glide, which reduces the risk of strained or torn muscles.

The combination of strengthening, cardiovascular, and stretching can be done in various ways. For example, we could do some weight lifting in the morning and some yoga at night. Or, perhaps a morning walk and some swimming in the afternoon. As long as we get these three exercise elements into our lives regularly, we will get what we need in movement.

What kind of exercise we get is up to us. We can choose what suits us and what works for us and decide when and where to do it. Some folks enjoy going to the gym and using the machines. Some folks want outdoor activities like jogging, swimming, or team sports. Some folks prefer to exercise in the privacy of their home. The internet can be an excellent resource for folks who enjoy following along with a video and watching an instructor. The options are many, and so are the benefits.

In short, our body needs to move to be healthy and strong. Moving our body will keep it in a state that we can enjoy. Not moving our body will result in losing our ability to live and move pain-free. So we say, "move it or lose it."

## Finding a Balance

Finding a balance between physical health and other areas of life is essential for health and wholeness. While physical health is undoubtedly important, it is just one aspect of holistic health, including mental, emotional, and spiritual health. Here are some tips for finding a balance between physical health and other areas of life:

- Set realistic goals: It is essential to set realistic goals for physical activity and nutrition that balance with other obligations and commitments. This can help prevent burnout and make you more likely to stick with your healthy habits.
- Practice self-care: Self-care involves taking time to prioritize your own needs and well-being. This can include engaging in activities that bring you joy and relaxation and taking care of your physical and emotional health.
- Build a support system: Social support can make it easier to maintain healthy habits and balance physical health and other areas of life. This can include friends, family, or support groups.
- Take breaks: Taking breaks from physical activity and work is essential, as overexertion can be detrimental to physical and mental health. Finding time for relaxation can help improve overall well-being.

Finding a balance between physical health and other areas of life is essential for overall well-being. Working with a holistic health provider and incorporating a range of practices and habits that support your holistic health is crucial for health and longevity.

## The Elephant Rope Parable as adapted by Jawahar Lalla

A gentleman was walking through an elephant camp and noticed that the elephants weren't being kept in cages or held by chains.

Only a small piece of rope tied to one of their legs was holding them back from escaping the camp. As the man gazed upon the elephants, he was completely confused about why they didn't just use their strength to break the rope and escape the camp. They could have quickly done so, but they didn't try to at all.

Curious to know the answer, he asked a trainer why the elephants were standing there and never tried to escape.

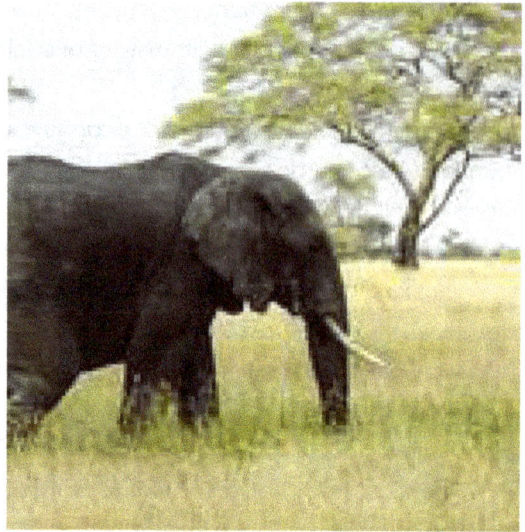

Image by Budz.McKenzie

The trainer replied, "When they are very young and much smaller, we use the same size rope to tie them, and, at that age, it's enough to hold them. As they grow up, they are conditioned to believe they cannot break away. They believe the rope can still hold them, so they never try to break free."

The only reason the elephants weren't breaking free and escaping from the camp was that, over time, they adopted the belief that it just wasn't possible.

The story of the elephants is metaphoric for life. Do you have an elephant mindset? Like the elephants, how many of us go through life hanging onto a belief (false) that we cannot do something simply because we failed at it once before? Every one of us can relate to this story. The feeling of having failed at something, and then over time, we began to believe that we are incapable of doing a particular thing. We accept this as the truth and limit ourselves to a confined world.

No matter how much the world tries to hold you back, always believe that you can and will be able to do what you set your mind to. You can achieve whatever you dream of in your life.

Assuming you can become successful (in whatever manner) is the most crucial step in achieving it. The false fears, obstacles, and challenges should not stop you from getting the success and happiness you deserve!

## Key Takeaways

This chapter covered components of physical fitness, the relationship between physical health and disease prevention, and the connection between physical and mental health. The chapter also explored holistic approaches to physical health, emphasizing the importance of finding balance in all areas of life.

## Questions For Reflection:

1. **How do I currently take care of my physical health?**

2. **Do I exercise? Which exercises do I want to try?**

3. **How can I bring more physical self-care into my daily life?**

*Take a Moment*

_____

_____

_____

_____

_____

_____

_____

_____

_____

_____

_____

_____

_____

_____

_____

In the next chapter, you will learn about the mental aspects of holistic health. We shall dive into the mind-body connection and provide great suggestions to improve mental health.

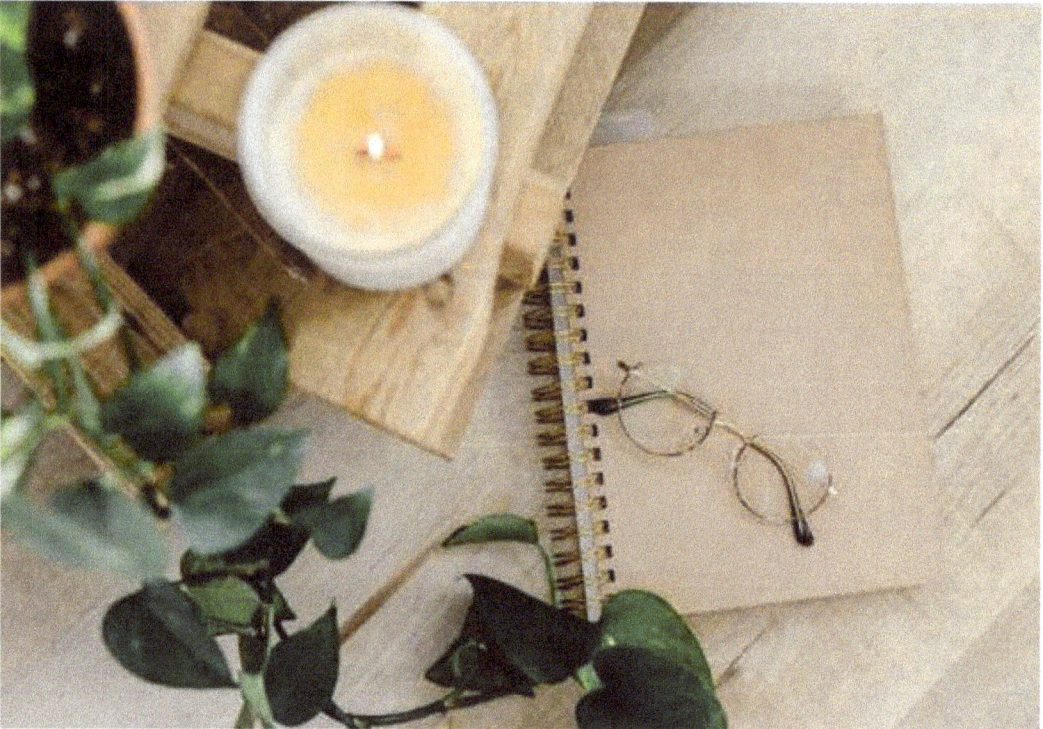

When mental health is compromised, it can have a wide range of adverse effects on physical fitness, relationships, work, and daily activities. The World Health Organization defines mental health disorder as "characterized by a clinically significant disturbance in an individual's cognition, emotional regulation or behavior. It is usually associate with distress or impairment in important areas of functioning."

Conditions such as depression and anxiety can cause physical symptoms such as fatigue and headaches and may negatively impact sleep and appetite. PTSD, eating disorders, bipolar disorder, and schizophrenia, among others, can significantly disrupt daily life and interfere with relationships and work and may also have physical manifestations.

It is crucial to prioritize and care for mental health through self-care practices, such as exercise, therapy, and spending time with loved ones. Seeking professional help through therapy or counseling can also be beneficial in managing stress and improving overall mental health.

Mental health is a key component of health and wellness and should be viewed as equally important as physical health. Taking care of one's mental health is critical to a healthy lifestyle and can positively impact all aspects of life.

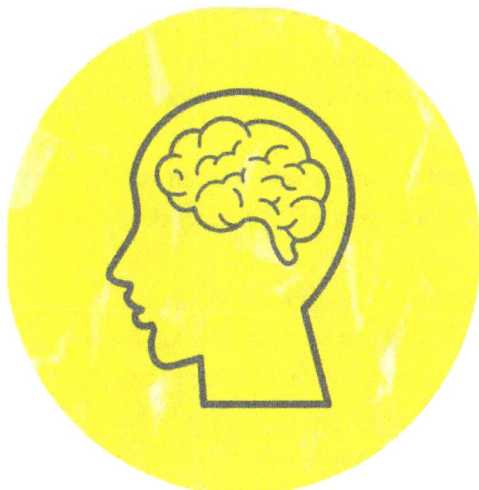

# Chapter Four: Mental Aspects of Holistic Health

*"It's important to point out that mental health is more about wellness rather than sickness."*
*-Matt Purcell*

## The Importance of Mental Health

Mental health is key to so many aspects of health. Mental health includes emotional, psychological, and social well-being and impacts how we think, feel, and act daily. Good mental health is essential for maintaining positive relationships, functioning at work or school, and living a fulfilling life.

## Changing Your Mindset about Your Health by Sharry

Did you know that how you think and talk about yourself could change how your body will respond? Changing how we see ourselves is a method used successfully for thousands of years as a part of healing by priests, shamans, yoga and meditation teachers, and healers who know and understand the connection between mind and body.

Recently, a branch of medicine called neuroscience has proven that mindset affects the body by using brain scans and chemical analysis of blood. By exposing a person to a particular stimulus, brain waves change, and chemical changes in blood composition are detected. Pain, pleasure, fear, comfort, and other emotions are just as much a part of our body as our bones and muscles. What we emotionally experience will determine the chemical composition of our blood and the effect it will have on our physical body.

You have the power to determine how you think and feel about yourself. You can make changes in your life. You can decide what and whom you want to expose yourself to, and by doing so, you can improve your health, energy, and relationships profoundly.

Human beings are, by nature, afraid of change. We adapt to our surroundings and circumstances and find it difficult, even terrifying, to change what has become familiar. Therefore, it may be wise to make slow and gradual changes and allow yourself time to adjust to one change before moving on to another. You cannot become a completely new person overnight, but over time, you will feel healthier, stronger, and more accessible in your body and overall life. Here are a few ideas to get you started.

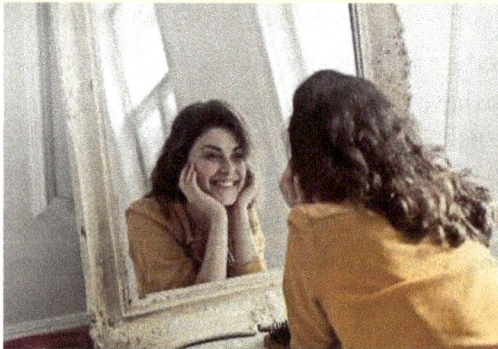

Begin by simply accepting yourself for who you are and how you feel. This is the most challenging step and is the basis for change. This step may involve a bruise to the ego, disappointment, or a feeling that you've let yourself and others down, but it is not valid and is the beginning of change. It would be best to become aware of yourself first to see what needs to change.

Take a good, long look at yourself in a mirror. Notice your hair color, eye color, and any spots or wrinkles on your face. Smile and see how that changes your look.

Next, take a look at your whole body. Clothed or unclothed, it's up to you. Notice how your body is shaped if it is large or small, short or tall. Do this without judging what it should be, and take note of what it is. Look at yourself with love. Love for the gift of life that you have been given. Love for the good things about your body.

Take note of how you feel. Where in your body are you feeling any pain or discomfort? Try not to run from it. Instead, feel and experience the sensations. This is part of you that you can control and manage more easily by changing your thoughts. For now, feel it and allow yourself to be aware of it. Remember that any changes you make in your thinking will affect how your body looks and feels. And how you see it. Wayne Dyer said, "When you change how you look at things, the things you look at change." These are some very profound and healing words.

Now, sit down and think about your living environment. Are you living with positive and supportive people? If you work, are you happy with your job and coworkers? Are you around people who like to tease or criticize you or people who lift you and inspire you? These outside influences are also huge in how you think and feel about yourself and how your body will feel. There is an expression, "Sticks and stones may break my bones, but words will never harm me." Not so. Broken bones will heal, but a broken spirit can stay with us forever. If you find yourself living and working around others who do not treat you well or speak ill of you or to you, it may be wise to detach yourself from them.

Separating yourself from others is one of the more difficult parts of changing your life, and if you need it, there are support groups that may help detach yourself from these hurtful influences. Most of us have a relative that fits into this category, and since we cannot choose our family, we can keep them at arm's length or love them from a distance. They often don't realize what they're doing is hurting you. Remember, you cannot control what others do or say, but you can control how you react to them.

Another influence on your thinking is what you expose yourself to on TV, movies, and social media. In this day and age, there are thousands of choices in TV shows and movies. Try to choose programming that makes you feel good. Avoid violence and crime shows. Our subconscious mind does not distinguish between something that happens to us directly or from something we see or hear about happening to someone else.

Have you noticed that when watching some action scene or a scene from a horror or suspense movie, your body seems to tense up? Your body thinks this is happening to you and is beginning the fight or flight response, releasing stress hormones, anticipating trouble, and preparing you to survive a dangerous situation. Repeatedly releasing these stress hormones can damage cells and cause pain and inflammation.

In repeated tests, participants were exposed to movies and videos depicting violence and abuse, and each time, their brain waves showed activity as if they were being hurt. Their blood tests showed elevated stress hormone levels just from watching. Be mindful of exposure to these visuals, especially the news. It's okay to keep up on current events, but keep it to a minimum.

Try reading books or watching videos about positive thinking and a positive outlook on life. The internet or the library is an excellent place to go for this. A few inspirational speakers/writers who helped me are Dr. Joe Dispenza, Dr. Bruce Lipton, Wayne Dyer, and Deepak Chopra. Listen to a few and follow the people who reach you. Everyone has a different way of speaking, and finding someone you can relate to will help you learn to think differently.

In my healing, I read and listened to many pastors and inspirational speakers. I am a follower of God, and I rely heavily on prayer and the knowledge that He is on my side and wants me to be well. Following a particular religion or spiritual path will be another helpful asset in your approach to wellness.

It is also helpful to post positive affirmations and words of encouragement around your house. Cut out positive words from magazines and tape them to doors and mirrors. Post pictures of happy people and happy moments. This constant visual will help you become familiar with the new thinking.

Tell yourself daily that you are getting better, healthier, and happier. For the most part, you are in control of your life and surroundings, and being in control is good medicine.

Our society has placed too much importance on how we should look. We are constantly being compared or comparing ourselves to the actors and the folks who are idolized on TV, in movies, and magazines. These people have been in makeup for hours, or their photos have been edited to make them look like the perfect person. They may wear girdles under their clothing to conceal loose or flabby places in their bodies. They are in costume. In real life, these folks also have moles, scars, warts, colored patches on their skin, and so on. They are real people under all that makeup.

All the marks on our bodies -- the warts, moles, scars, and such -- indicate that we have lived and are authentic. Some spots are genetic, while others are marks from events we have experienced: accidents, surgeries, illnesses, and even self-induced harm. Whatever the reason, whatever the source of these marks-- embrace them as part of the whole, authentic you. Accepting these marks will help ease your feelings about them and reduce your stress levels, which will be another part of the puzzle in healing your body, mind, and spirit. (I remember a moment in my early 60s when I developed "bat wings" under my arms and laughed at the saggy skin. And still do.)

Laughter is another excellent tool for easing stress and improving your outlook on life. Laughter induces feel-good hormones and puts the stress hormones in check.

It doesn't have to be loud and gut-busting; even a simple chuckle is enough to do the trick. Try looking in the mirror and laughing. It may seem stiff initially, but it will become natural over time. Remember, you are learning, and learning takes time.

These are a few ideas and bits of information that may help you take the first steps in becoming healthier and happier. You may find other strategies that work for you, and that's great. Your health and happiness are personal things you, and you alone, are in control of. You have the power. Use it.

## MENTAL HEALTH FIRST STEPS

- MAKE TIME FOR ACTIVITIES YOU ENJOY
- CHALLENGE NEGATIVE THOUGHTS AND SELF-TALK
- SET ACHIEVABLE GOALS
- FOCUS ON YOUR STRENGTHS
- SURROUND YOURSELF WITH POSITIVE PEOPLE
- SEEK HELP WHEN NEEDED

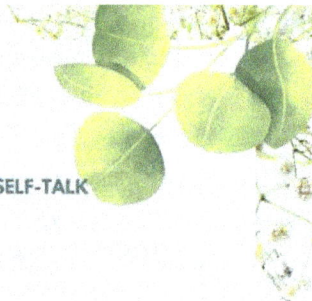

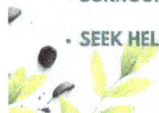

## Developing Positive Coping Strategies

Positive coping strategies are any actions or behaviors that help an individual manage and reduce stress in their life in a way that isn't harmful or detrimental. Developing positive coping strategies involves identifying and utilizing healthy outlets that help manage stress and build resilience. Here are some examples of positive coping strategies:

- Exercise: Physical activity helps release endorphins, promoting happiness and well-being.
- Mindfulness: Practicing mindfulness can help individuals learn to accept and tolerate difficult emotions without judgment and cope with stressful situations healthily.
- Social Support: Spending time with friends and family members who offer positive emotional support can help build resilience and reduce stress.
- Relaxation Techniques: Deep breathing, yoga, and meditation can help induce calm and relaxation, which can be particularly helpful during stressful situations.
- Creative Outlets: Engaging in hobbies or creative activities, such as painting or writing, can provide a sense of accomplishment and help manage stress.
- Professional Help: Talking to a therapist, coach, or counselor can help individuals develop healthier coping mechanisms and better manage stress.

Positive coping strategies are essential for managing stress and building resilience in difficult situations. Individuals can improve their health and lead a happier, more fulfilling life by identifying and utilizing healthy coping mechanisms.

### Creating a Sense of Purpose

Creating a purpose can be vital in achieving personal and professional fulfillment. Here are a few strategies that can help:

- Identify Your Values: Understanding what you value most in life can give you a sense of direction and clarity when creating a sense of purpose. List your core values and identify ways to apply them to your daily life.
- Set Goals: Setting achievable, meaningful goals can help create a sense of purpose and direction. Make a list of short-term and long-term goals, and work towards those goals consistently.
- Find Meaning in Your Work: If you can find meaning and purpose in your work, it can have a positive impact on your health and well-being. Identify ways your work positively impacts others, and try to focus on those aspects of your job.
- Connect with Others: Building positive relationships and finding a sense of community can create a sense of purpose. Look for ways to connect with others who share your interests and values.
- Give Back: Volunteering or engaging in other types of service can provide a sense of purpose and fulfillment. Look for opportunities to give back to your community or those in need.

Creating a sense of purpose involves identifying what matters most and finding meaningful ways to apply those values to your life. By focusing on your values, setting goals, finding meaning in your work, connecting with others, and giving back, you can develop a stronger sense of purpose and achieve greater fulfillment.

In our experience, many clients are dissatisfied with their work and home life. It is like a light switch when we tell them they can find meaning and fulfillment in any job. All they have to do is change how they think about what they are doing. For example, they may be unhappy as a data entry clerk, and finding something to enjoy about doing that every day may be challenging. Yet they enjoy their interactions with coworkers. So they look forward to work as the opportunity to interact with people they enjoy. A simple change in how you think about what you are doing can create a sense of purpose.

## A Sense of Purpose by Sharry

How do you feel at the end of the day? Are you tired from working? Did you accomplish something? If so, isn't that a wonderful feeling?

When we are ill for a long time or injured and recovering, it can be challenging to do the things we like to do. It cannot be easy to just take care of ourselves. Even the little things like bathing or preparing something to eat can be exhausting. It is tempting to stay in bed. Initially, we need the extra rest to let our body heal. However, prolonged bedrest or being idle for too long can harm physical and mental health.

Human beings were designed to move and do things -- to work, to create, to be up and around on our feet daily. Most of us have a job or are taking care of our home and family. That can be our purpose. When we are not working, or our families are grown and no longer need our daily sustenance, then what do we do? We find another purpose. That purpose may be volunteering at a church food bank or working with children. Volunteering is a beautiful way to experience meaning and, at the same time, help someone else.

Finding a purpose is a massive part of our recovery if we cannot get out of the house or recover from a prolonged health situation. When we can do something, however small, it lets our brain send out feel-good hormones like dopamine. Feel-good

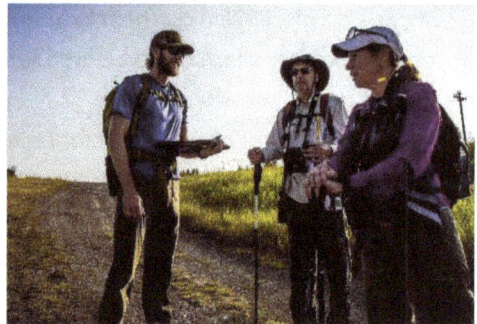

Image by GlacierNPS

hormones help us want to do something again because it feels good. Feeling good leads to improved health.

When we give in and do nothing, our brain doesn't send out the feel-good hormones. Instead, the brain gets sluggish and a little foggy. We lose interest in life and the things we used to enjoy. Depression can be the result. Coming out of depression can be challenging and takes time. We can avoid depression by finding a purpose and staying busy and engaged.

On a personal note, I had surgery that left me exhausted and in lots of chronic pain. This went on for months, and several doctors told me nothing could be done, that I was getting old before my time, and to get used to it. I chose another path.

I began walking around the house at first. Then, I started doing a little light cleaning, resumed my yoga practice, and began to read, study, and write. I learned to cook, care for my yard, and change my mindset from "disabled" to "getting back in the game." This took time and effort. At times, I felt like giving in and accepting being homebound. I did spend a lot of time lying down, but I got up and did something every day. I had about 3 hours of physical activity before the screaming, burning pain set in. But until then, I did things. I cleaned something. I cooked a meal. I picked some weeds. I did daily yoga. Then, when the pain set in, I hit the couch with my narcotic meds. The next day, I got up and did more.

Instinctively, I knew that this was part of my healing and recovery. I knew that one day, I would be well again. I told my son, "I'm gonna get off this couch one day." And I did. My body will never be quite the same, as the surgery did not work, and I have to be careful how much I do, how long, and how often. But I am working again, and I have a positive mental attitude.

Having a purpose for myself led to a positive mindset and a healthier body. It is not only possible, it is free. But you have to show up for yourself, and when you do, you will be glad you did.

The choice is yours. Give in and do nothing, or get up and live.

## Mental Health Practices to Improve Cognition

Several mental health practices have been shown to improve cognitive performance.

Here are a few examples:

- Mindfulness and meditation can improve working memory, attention, and cognitive flexibility. Practicing mindfulness and meditation involves directing your attention to the present moment and accepting it without judgment.
- Regular exercise has been shown to improve cognitive function, including memory, attention, and executive function. Exercise promotes the growth of new neurons and the release of neurotransmitters that support cognitive function.
- Sleep is essential for cognitive function, allowing the brain to consolidate memories and process new information. Chronic sleep deprivation has been linked to impaired cognitive function.
- Cognitive Behavioral Therapy (CBT) is a type of talk therapy shown to improve cognitive function and reduce symptoms of anxiety and depression. CBT helps individuals identify negative thinking patterns and develop more positive and adaptive ways of thinking.
- Social support from friends and family can improve cognitive performance and reduce the adverse effects of stress on the brain. Social interaction promotes the release of oxytocin, a hormone associated with positive social behavior.

Several mental health practices can help improve cognitive performance. You can improve your cognitive health and overall well-being by incorporating mindfulness meditation, exercise, adequate sleep, cognitive behavioral therapy, and social support into your routine.

## Mental Health Prevents Chronic Disease

Mental health plays a crucial role in preventing chronic diseases. Poor mental health can increase the risk of developing chronic diseases, such as heart disease and diabetes, making managing these conditions more difficult. In addition, many chronic diseases are accompanied by mental health issues, such as depression and anxiety.

One way mental health can help prevent chronic diseases is by promoting healthy behaviors. Individuals with good mental health are more likely to engage in healthy behaviors, such as exercising regularly and eating a healthy diet.

Another way that mental health can help prevent chronic diseases is by reducing stress levels. Chronic stress has been linked to an increased risk of developing chronic conditions, such as heart disease and diabetes. Individuals can reduce their risk of developing chronic diseases by managing stress through stress-reducing techniques, such as mindfulness meditation or cognitive behavioral therapy.

Mental health treatment can help individuals manage chronic diseases more effectively. Individuals with chronic diseases are more likely to experience depression and anxiety, making it more challenging to manage their condition. By addressing these mental health issues, individuals can improve their overall health outcomes and better manage their chronic disease.

Overall, mental health plays an essential role in preventing chronic diseases. By promoting healthy behaviors, reducing stress levels, and providing mental health treatment, individuals can reduce their risk of developing chronic diseases or better manage their condition.

## The Importance of Screenings and Check-ups

While regular check-ups and screenings are often associated with physical health, they are also crucial for maintaining good mental health. Here are some reasons why mental health screenings and check-ups are essential:

- Early Detection: Mental health disorders are easiest to treat when they are caught early.
- Preventative Care: Mental health screenings can be used to assess an individual's risk for developing a mental health disorder. Individuals may benefit from preventive care, such as stress-reducing techniques or therapy.
- Improved Quality of Life: Mental health screenings and check-ups can improve quality of life by identifying and treating mental health issues that may be impacting an individual's daily life.
- Reduced Stigma: Mental health screenings and check-ups can help reduce the stigma associated with mental health by making it a routine part of healthcare.
- Integrated Care: Holistic providers offer integrated care, including physical and mental health services. Regular check-ups and screenings can ensure that individuals

receive integrated care for all aspects of their health.

Regular mental health screenings and check-ups are essential to maintaining good mental health. By identifying and treating mental health issues early, individuals can improve their quality of life and reduce the impact that mental health issues have on their daily lives.

## Reduce Mental Health Condition Risk

There are several ways to reduce the risk of developing mental health conditions. Here are some examples:

- Exercise: Regular exercise has been shown to reduce the risk of developing mental health conditions, such as depression and anxiety. Exercise promotes the release of endorphins, which are natural mood boosters.
- Healthy Diet: A healthy diet can help reduce the risk of developing, or impact of, mental health conditions. A diet rich in fruits, vegetables, and lean protein can provide the nutrients the brain needs to function correctly.
- Stress Management: Stress has been linked to the development of mental health conditions. Effective stress management techniques, such as meditation or deep breathing, can reduce the impact of stress on the body and mind.
- Social Support: Social support from family and friends can reduce the risk of developing mental health conditions by providing a sense of belonging and connectedness.

- Sleep: Getting enough sleep is also crucial for maintaining good mental health. Lack of sleep can lead to depression, anxiety, and other mental health conditions.

Taking care of one's physical and emotional health through regular exercise, healthy eating, stress management, social support, and getting enough sleep can reduce the risk of developing mental health conditions.

Since mental and physical health are so intertwined, the same suggestions for reducing risks for one works for the other. This makes it simple to learn and incorporate into our daily lives.

## The Mental and Physical Health Connection

There is a strong connection between physical health and mental health. The two are closely linked and can significantly impact each other. Here are some examples of the relationship between physical health and mental health:

- Chronic Physical Conditions: People with chronic physical conditions, such as diabetes or heart disease, are more likely to experience mental health issues, such as depression or anxiety.
- Lifestyle Factors: Lifestyle factors like diet and exercise can impact physical and mental health. Eating a healthy diet and engaging in regular activity can improve physical health and have a positive impact on mental health as well.
- Stress: Stress can harm both physical and mental health. Chronic stress can lead to physical health issues, such as high blood

pressure, and can also lead to mental health issues, such as anxiety and depression.

- **Sleep:** Poor sleep can harm both physical and mental health. Lack of sleep can lead to physical health issues, such as obesity and diabetes, and mental health issues, such as depression and anxiety.
- **Brain Chemicals:** Brain chemicals, such as serotonin and dopamine, play a role in physical and mental health. Imbalances in these chemicals can lead to both physical and mental health issues.

Taking care of physical and mental health is vital for a well-balanced life. Being physically active, eating a healthy diet, managing stress, getting enough sleep, and seeking professional help are just a few ways to promote good physical and mental health. Again, what works for one tends to work for the other.

## Benefits of Physical Activity for Mental Health

Physical activity has numerous benefits for mental health. Here are some of the help:

- **Reduced Symptoms of Depression and Anxiety:** Regular physical activity has been shown to reduce symptoms of depression and anxiety. Exercise releases endorphins, which are natural mood boosters and can reduce the levels of stress hormones in the body.
- **Improved Self-Esteem:** Physical activity can improve self-esteem, especially regarding body image. Exercise has been linked to improved body image and increased confidence in one's abilities.

- **Reduced Risk of Cognitive Decline:** Regular physical activity has been linked to a reduced risk of cognitive decline later in life. Exercise can improve cognitive function, including memory, attention, and executive function.
- **Improved Sleep:** Exercise can also improve sleep, essential to mental health. Regular physical activity can help regulate sleep patterns and enhance the quality of sleep.
- **Stress Reduction:** Regular physical activity can also help manage stress levels, which can significantly impact mental health. Exercise can help relieve tension and stress, promoting relaxation and well-being.

Physical activity has numerous mental health benefits, including reducing symptoms of depression and anxiety, improving self-esteem, reducing the risk of cognitive decline, improving sleep, and reducing stress. Therefore, incorporating regular physical activity into daily life can immensely benefit mental health.

## Integrating Mental Health Practices

Integrating mental health practices with other aspects of holistic health is an essential approach to health and wellness. The holistic health approach recognizes that physical, mental, and social well-being are interconnected and interdependent. Therefore, addressing mental health concerns involves integrating mental health with other aspects of health, such as physical health, nutrition, and social support.

Here are some ways mental health practices can be integrated with other aspects of holistic health:

- **Exercise:** Incorporating exercise into mental health treatment can improve mood, reduce symptoms of anxiety and depression, and provide a sense of accomplishment that can boost self-esteem.

- **Nutrition:** A healthy diet can benefit both physical and mental health. For example, foods containing certain nutrients, such as omega-3 fatty acids, have been linked to improved brain function and reduced symptoms of depression and anxiety. Therefore, incorporating nutrition counseling and education into mental health treatment can be beneficial.

- **Social Support:** Integrating social interventions, such as group therapy or peer support groups, can provide a sense of community and belonging that can be helpful for people struggling with mental health concerns.

- **Complementary and Alternative Medicine:** Holistic health approaches often include complementary and alternative medicine (CAM), such as acupuncture, massage, and meditation. Incorporating CAM practices into mental health treatment can provide an additional tool for managing symptoms and promoting overall health.

Integrating mental health practices with other aspects of holistic health can provide a comprehensive approach to promoting mental health and well-being. It recognizes the interconnectedness of physical, mental, and social health and can provide a more practical approach to addressing mental health concerns.

We have holistic practitioners on our online platform, Holistic Bodyworks Online, (https://holisticbodyworksonline.community) who can help to provide a plan of action that includes the different aspects of holistic health. A more holistic approach makes healing from a mental or physical illness attainable.

## Finding Balance

Finding a balance between mental health and other areas of life is crucial for health and wellness. It is essential to recognize that mental health is interconnected with other areas of life, such as physical health, social relationships, work, and personal interests. Focusing only on one area of life can lead to neglecting other areas, impacting mental health.

Below are some strategies for finding a balance between mental health and other areas of life:

- **Practice Self-Care:** Practicing self-care is essential for maintaining mental wellness. Whether reading a book, going for a walk, or engaging in a hobby, taking time for oneself can help alleviate stress and promote positive mental health.

- **Set Healthy Boundaries:** It is essential to set limits and boundaries in all areas of life, including work, relationships, and personal time. This can involve saying no to additional responsibilities when feeling overwhelmed and setting boundaries with others to prevent overextending oneself.

- **Build a Support Network:** Having social support is essential for mental health. Building relationships with family, friends, or colleagues can provide emotional support and help reduce stress.

- **Maintaining a Healthy Lifestyle:** A healthy lifestyle should include regular exercise, healthy eating habits, and getting enough sleep, which can also help promote good mental health.

- **Seek Professional Help:** If you are struggling with mental health concerns, seeking help from a mental health professional can be beneficial. Cognitive-behavioral therapy and mindfulness can help individuals develop coping strategies and better manage stress.

Finding a balance between mental health and other areas of life requires intentional effort and prioritization. Prioritizing self-care, setting healthy boundaries, building a support network, maintaining a healthy lifestyle, and seeking professional help when needed can all contribute to achieving balance and promoting mental health.

### The Owl and the Chimpanzee by Jo Camacho

The owl and the chimpanzee went to sea
In a beautiful boat called The Mind
The owl was sensible, clever and smart
The chimp was a little behind
The owl made decisions, based on fact
And knew where to steer its ship
The chimp reacted a little too fast
And often the boat would tip
The waves would come and crash aboard
The chimp would start to cry
Large tears would roll right down his face
Afraid that he would die
The chimp and the owl would wrestle at night
When the world was quiet and still
The chimp would jump up and rock the boat
And the boat would start to fill
Then the owl stepped in and grabbed a pail
And started to empty it out
And the chimp would start to get quite cross
And would often scream and shout
The battle continued night after night
Until the chimp started to see
That if it let the owl take control
A more peaceful night it would be

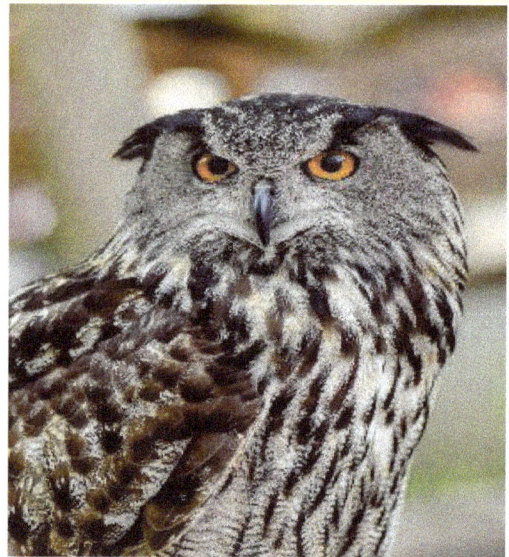

Image by Mathias Appel

This poem by clinical hypnotherapist and psychotherapist Jo Camacho beautifully articulates the internal battle many of us face when the more primitive part of our brain (the chimp brain) takes control. The wise owl within all of us is seen here fighting with the chimp, who seems determined to make the situation worse despite its fears of the crisis worsening.

This poem teaches us that internal conflict is normal and human. If we learn to control our primitive, scared brain more often and listen to our inner owl, we'll enjoy a more peaceful journey.

## Changing Mindsets to Achieve Highest Potential by Stephanie

Believe you can succeed, and you will!

How do you develop the power of belief? Think success, don't think failure. At work, in your home, substitute failure thinking for success thinking. When you face a difficult situation, think, "I'll win," not "I'll probably lose." When thinking of changing health habits, think "I can do it," never "I can't." Let the master thought, "I will succeed," dominate your thinking process. Thinking success conditions the mind to create plans that produce success. Thinking failure does the exact opposite. Failure thinking conditions the mind to feel other thoughts that make a failure.

Remind yourself regularly that you are better than you think you are. Successful people are not supermen/women. Success does not require a super-intellect. Nor is there anything mystical about ordinary folks who have developed a belief in themselves and what they do. Never sell yourself short.

Believe Big. The size of your belief determines the size of your success. Think of little goals and expect little achievements. Think big dreams and win big success. Big ideas and plans are often more straightforward — indeed no more difficult — than small ideas and techniques.

Cure yourself of excusitis, the failure disease!

"But my health isn't good."

"I don't feel good."

"I've got such-and-such wrong with me."

Refuse to talk about your poor health. The more you talk about an ailment, even the common cold, the worse it seems. Talking about lousy health is like putting fertilizer on weeds. Besides, talking about your health is a bad habit. Success-minded people defeat the natural tendency to talk about their "bad" health. One may get a little sympathy but doesn't get respect and loyalty by being a chronic complainer.

Refuse to worry about your health. Be genuinely grateful that your health is as good as it is. There's an old saying worth repeating often: "I felt sorry for myself because I had ragged shoes until I met a man who had no feet." Instead of complaining about "not feeling good," it's far better to be glad you are as healthy as you are. Being grateful for your health is a powerful vaccination against developing new aches, pains, and illnesses.

Remind yourself often, "It's better to wear out than rust out." Life is yours to enjoy. Please don't waste it. Don't pass up living by thinking yourself into a hospital bed.

When you're alone with your thoughts — driving in your car or eating alone — recall pleasant, positive experiences. This boosts confidence. It gives you that "I-sure-feel-good" feeling. It helps keep your body functioning right, too.

Just before you go to sleep, focus on good thoughts. Count your blessings. Recall the many good things you have to be thankful for: your wife or husband, your children, your friends, and your health.

Recall the good things you saw people do today. Recall your little victories and accomplishments, and explain why you are glad to be alive.

Use big, positive, cheerful words and phrases to describe your feelings. When someone asks, "How do you feel today?" and you respond with an "I'm tired (I have a headache, I don't feel so good)," you make yourself feel worse. Practice answering like this: "Just wonderful, thanks, and you?" or say "Great" or "Fine" with enthusiasm!

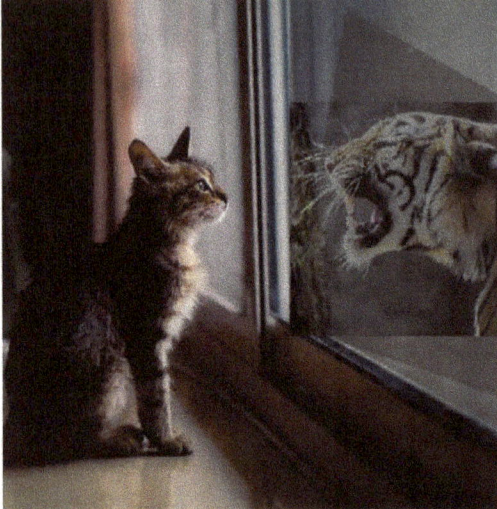

Believe!! When you believe, your mind finds ways to do it. Belief releases creative powers. Disbelief puts the brakes on.

Give yourself a pep talk several times daily. Build a "sell-yourself-to-yourself" commercial. Remind yourself at every opportunity that you're a healthy, energetic, and fit person.

Make your environment make you successful!

Be environmental-conscious. Make your environment work for you, not against you. Make your home a sanctuary to nurture you.

Don't let suppressive forces — the negative, you-can't-do-it people — make you think "defeat." Don't let small-thinking people hold you back. Jealous people want to see you stumble. Please don't give them that satisfaction. Get your advice from successful people. Throw thought poison out of your environment. Avoid gossip. Talk about people, but stay on the positive side.

Get plenty of psychological sunshine. Circulate in new groups. Discover new and stimulating things to do. Get in the action habit!

Use a mechanical approach to accomplish simple but sometimes unpleasant business and household chores. Rather than think about the undesirable features of the task, jump right in and get going without much deliberation.

Next, use the mechanical way to create ideas, map plans, solve problems, and do other work requiring top mental performance. Rather than wait for the spirit to move you, sit down and carry your energy. Just start the process without waiting until the conditions are perfect. They never will be.

Remember, ideas alone won't bring success. Ideas have value only when you act upon them! Use action to cure fear and gain confidence. Do what you fear and fear disappears. Just try it and see. Think in terms of NOW. Tomorrow, next week, later, and similar words often are synonymous with the failure word, NEVER. Be an "I'll start right now" kind of person.

## Key Takeaways

This chapter provided an overview of the mental aspect of holistic health, highlighting the importance of mental health in maintaining overall wellness and well-being. It covered mental health components, the relationship between mental health and disease prevention, and the connection between physical health and mental health.

The chapter also explored holistic approaches to mental health, emphasizing the importance of finding balance in all areas of life.

## Exercise for building confidence and destroying fear:

1. Isolate your fear, pin it down, and determine what you are afraid of. Ponder and write what you come up with.

2. Then, take action. There is some action for any kind of fear. Write down a goal for destroying fear that requires effort.

# Questions For Reflection:

1. **How do I currently take care of my mental health?**

2. **Do I exercise my mind daily?**

3. **What can I add to my daily routine to exercise my mind?**

4. **How can I bring mental self-care into my everyday life?**

## Take a Moment

_____

_____

_____

_____

_____

_____

_____

_____

_____

_____

_____

_____

_____

_____

_____

_____

_____

_____

_____

_____

_____

_____

_____

_____

_____

_____

_____

_____

In the next chapter, you will learn about the social aspects of holistic health, how to build your support network for social interactions, and the importance of not leaving out the social part when striving to embrace a simply holistic lifestyle.

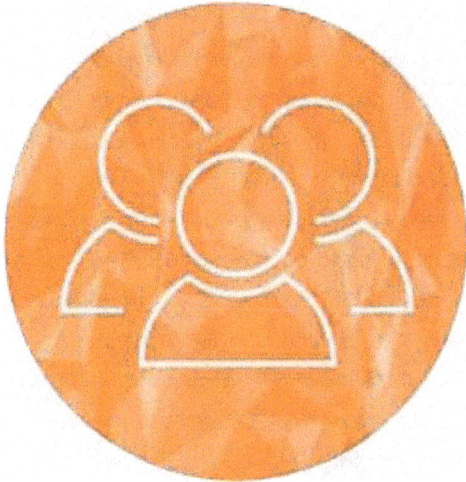

# Chapter Five: Social Aspects of Holistic Health

*"What mental health needs are more sunlight, more candor, and more unashamed conversation."*
*-Glenn Close*

## Social Aspects of Holistic Health

Social health involves an individual's relationships, connections, and interactions with others in their environment. Studies have shown that social support and connections are crucial for maintaining and improving health and that social support can help individuals cope with stress, build resilience, and improve mental health. Additionally, socially connected people are more likely to engage in healthy behaviors.

One way social support can be fostered is by creating social networks. Social networks can be created in numerous ways, such as joining clubs or groups that align with a person's interests or volunteering in the community. Social networks can be especially beneficial for older adults who may experience social isolation and loneliness.

Another critical aspect of social health is the environmental factors influencing health, such as access to healthcare, education, employment opportunities, and safe living conditions. Addressing these environmental factors can improve health outcomes for individuals and communities.

It is also important to note that societal attitudes and beliefs toward different groups of people can impact social health. Discrimination and stigmatization can negatively impact social health, leading to isolation and limited resource access.

Overall, addressing social health is an essential aspect of holistic health, and efforts should be made to improve social connections and address social determinants of health for individuals and communities.

## The Importance of Social Aspects

Holistic health recognizes that social factors, such as relationships, community involvement, and support networks can significantly impact one's physical, emotional, and spiritual well-being.

The importance of social aspects in holistic health lies in their ability to provide individuals with a sense of belonging, purpose, and support. Relationships with family, friends, and community members can help individuals stay connected and provide emotional support during difficult times. Social support can also help individuals deal with stress and reduce the risks of depression and anxiety.

Holistic health recognizes that social isolation and loneliness can exacerbate health problems and impede recovery. Studies show that individuals who report high levels of social support have better cardiovascular health, more robust immune systems, and lower levels of inflammation than those who lack social support.

Social interactions are an essential component of holistic health. Engaging in healthy relationships, connecting with others, and building social support networks are critical strategies for achieving balance and improving well-being. Holistic health recognizes that social factors are integral to one's health and encourages individuals to prioritize social connections and community involvement in their self-care efforts.

## The Social Dimension

The social dimension refers to an individual's social relationships and connectivity with others, including family, friends, and community. It also includes a sense of belonging, purpose, and support from social networks. The social dimension is a significant component of holistic health because it can positively impact an individual's physical, emotional, and spiritual well-being.

Strong social relationships and networks provide individuals with a support system during times of stress or hardship, help to reduce the risk of depression or anxiety and improve cardiovascular health, immunity, and inflammation levels. On the other hand, social isolation, loneliness, and lack of social support are pervasive health risks that can lead to adverse health outcomes, including morbidity and mortality. Thus, incorporating social strategies, such as community involvement and building social support networks, is crucial to achieving and maintaining optimal health.

Socializing is a basic human need for all of us. We are naturally gregarious creatures, which means we need each other to survive and thrive. Interactions between people generate an energy that connects, heals, and restores. Without this human interaction, we waste away.

In the early 1900s, many children and babies were homeless, without parents or anyone to care for them. Orphanages were created to give these little ones a home and get them off the street. However, there were not enough workers to care for the children. The workers had barely enough time to feed and bathe the babies and put them back into their cribs. During this time, many infants died within their first year, and the ones that lived were often mentally challenged or dwarfed from malnourishment. It became apparent to doctors that social interaction is crucial for children to live and grow into healthy adults. When more staff was added and more time was spent with the babies, their health and life expectancy improved. The need for this interaction doesn't stop there.

Adults also need social interaction. Engaging with others stimulates our brain to think, react, create, remember, and release our feel-good hormones.

When we are ill for an extended period or recovering from an injury or surgery, we need human interaction to help us heal. We need company and visitors. We need to know someone is there for us. Not everyone can engage with a friend or family member who is not up to par. People who cannot, will tend to stay away, not that they don't care but because they don't have what it takes to be a caregiver or nurturing friend. So it would seem that when these friends stop coming around, we have been abandoned and left to our fate. That's where volunteers and home health workers shine. They are people who have the nurturing personality and the caring heart that we need to recover. They are healing heroes.

In short, having someone to hear us and enjoy being with us can be life-saving. If we are homebound, we now have the blessing of social media and FaceTime calls. And if we can get out of the house, there are social gatherings, adult and senior classes, recreation centers, or volunteer opportunities. We don't have to be alone or isolated. We can reach out, and someone will be there. But we have to take that first step. Someone is out there for you. Give them, and yourself, a chance.

## Social Support Networks

Social support networks can significantly impact an individual's social health. Here are some ways in which social support networks can affect social health:

- Emotional support: Social support networks can provide emotional support to individuals during stressful or difficult situations. Having a supportive and caring social network can

help individuals cope with challenges and improve their overall emotional well-being.

- Sense of belonging: Social support networks can contribute to an individual's sense of belonging and provide a sense of purpose and identity. A sense of belonging can enhance an individual's social health by reducing feelings of isolation and loneliness.

- Self-esteem: Social support networks can also contribute to an individual's self-esteem and confidence in social situations. Individuals who have supportive networks tend to be more confident in themselves and their social interactions, leading to better social health.

On the other hand, a lack of social support networks can negatively impact social health. Individuals lacking social support may feel isolated disconnected from their community, and struggle with loneliness and low self-esteem.

Social support networks are crucial in shaping an individual's social health. Building and maintaining strong social connections with family, friends, and community can lead to a more fulfilling and enriched social life, contributing to overall wellness.

## SOCIAL HEALTH FIRST STEPS
- MAINTAIN A WORK-LIFE BALANCE
- SPEND TIME WITH FAMILY AND FRIENDS
- PARTICIPATE IN SOCIAL ACTIVITIES
- SET REACHABLE GOALS, THEN CELEBRATE WHEN YOU REACH THEM
- FIND HEALTHY NETWORKS TO BE INVOLVED IN

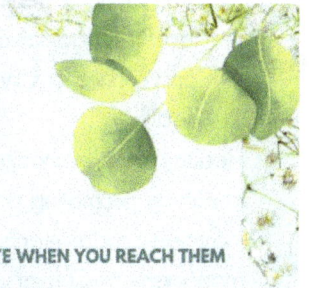

## Lifestyle Choices

While lifestyle choices can affect overall health, including physical and mental health, they can also impact social health. Here are a few ways in which lifestyle choices can affect social health:

- Social settings: Lifestyle choices such as drinking, smoking, or drug use can negatively impact social interactions. Excessive indulgence in negative behaviors can lead to social isolation, exclusion, or disconnection from social groups.

- Health behaviors: Engaging in healthy lifestyle behaviors such as regular exercise and a balanced diet can lead to a healthier body and mind. Additionally, these healthier behaviors can lead to social settings that promote health and well-being, enabling individuals to connect with others who share similar healthy beliefs and behaviors.

- Time management: Engaging in certain lifestyle behaviors, such as overworking, excessive use of social media, or irregular sleeping patterns can significantly impact time management. These behaviors can lead to a lack of time for social interactions and connections, negatively impacting social health.

Healthy lifestyle choices can improve social health by promoting positive behaviors, increasing social interactions, and better time management. Conversely, engaging in unhealthy lifestyles can lead to social isolation and disconnection.

## Strategies for Promoting Social Health

Promoting social health and improving social support networks can be achieved by implementing several strategies. Here are some strategies for promoting social health and improving social support networks:

- Participate in social activities: A great way to promote social health is to participate in social activities such as sports, clubs, library or church activities, or community service. Participating in these activities allows individuals to meet new people, expand their social networks, and engage in enjoyable hobbies.

Educational and training programs: Institutions and businesses can offer educational and training programs, such as skill-building workshops or social interaction training, to enhance social skills, improve communication, and support healthy relationships.

- Build community support groups: Community support groups offer a space for individuals to come together, share their experiences, and offer emotional support to each other. Mental health support groups, substance abuse recovery groups, and social skills support groups are just a few of the many community support groups available.

- Develop and nurture social relationships: To promote social health develop and encourage social relationships with family, friends, or colleagues at work. Maintaining these relationships can provide emotional support during times of need, promote positive behaviors, and foster a sense of belonging and connectedness within one's social world.

Engaging in social health and improving social support networks is crucial for emotional and mental well-being. By implementing various strategies, individuals and communities can enhance social health by encouraging participation in social activities, offering educational programs, building community support groups, and nurturing social relationships.

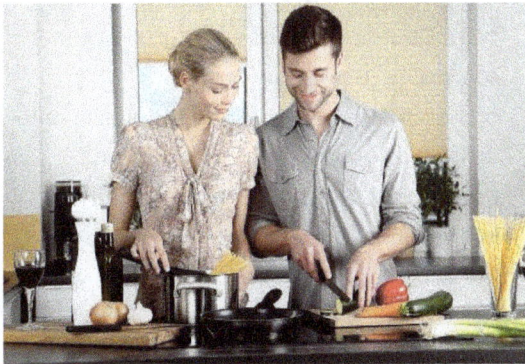

Image by Werner Heiber

## Engaging in Community Activities

Engaging in community activities is an excellent strategy for promoting social health. Community activities allow individuals to connect with others, develop social skills, and form meaningful relationships. Here are some more strategies that can help promote social health through community engagement:

- **Participate in community events:** Communities and community gathering centers host various events, such as festivals, concerts, and fairs -- all open to the public. Attending these events can provide opportunities to meet new people, engage in new experiences, and build connections.

- **Join community groups:** Communities often have various groups focused on interests such as arts, sports, volunteerism, or social justice. Joining one of these groups can offer individuals the chance to develop new friendships, share experiences, and engage in activities they enjoy.

- **Participate in community service:** Community service opportunities provide a way to contribute to society while connecting with others. Serving meals at a food bank, building homes for people experiencing homelessness, or cleaning up a local park are just a few examples of community service opportunities that can promote social health.

- **Volunteer with community organizations:** Organizations such as schools, churches, and non-profit organizations rely heavily on volunteers to perform various tasks. Volunteering can provide an opportunity to interact with others and build connections while contributing to one's community.

Engaging in community activities is a valuable strategy for social health. It allows individuals to connect with others, develop social skills, and form meaningful relationships. When individuals are engaged in community activities and service, they are more likely to feel a sense of belonging, connectedness, and purpose, leading to positive social outcomes.

## Encouraging Positive Interactions

Encouraging positive communication and interactions is an essential strategy for promoting social health. Positive communication and interactions can help individuals form meaningful relationships, develop social skills, and contribute to a sense of belonging. Here are some strategies that can help promote positive communication and interactions and contribute to social health:

- **Active listening:** Active listening involves giving full attention to the person speaking and responding in a way that shows comprehension and interest. Active listening in conversations can promote positive communication and interactions.

- **Respectful communication:** Communicating in a manner that is respectful of the other person's opinions, feelings, and beliefs can promote positive interactions and build healthy relationships.

- **Positive reinforcement:** Positive feedback and encouragement can help reinforce positive communication and interactions and promote healthy relationships.

- **Conflict resolution:** Encouraging individuals to address conflicts respectfully and constructively can help promote positive communication and interactions and reduce negative feelings and misunderstandings.

- **Build empathy:** Seeing things from another's perspective, and showing compassion, and understanding can promote positive communication, interactions, and healthy relationships.

Encouraging positive communication and interactions is an essential strategy for promoting social health. Active listening, respectful communication, positive reinforcement, conflict resolution, and building empathy are all important elements that can contribute to positive social interactions and help develop healthy relationships.

## Developing Social Skills

Social skills enable individuals to interact effectively with others, positively express themselves, and build meaningful relationships. Here are some strategies that can help promote the development of social skills and contribute to social health:

- **Encourage participation in social activities:** Encouraging individuals to engage in social activities, such as sports teams, clubs, or community groups, can provide opportunities for developing social skills and building relationships.

- **Practice active listening:** Practicing active listening involves giving full attention to the person speaking and responding in a way that shows comprehension and interest. By practicing active listening, individuals can develop interpersonal communication skills, contributing to positive social interactions.

- **Offer positive feedback:** Offering positive feedback and support can help individuals feel more comfortable and confident in social situations, promoting social skills development.

- **Build skills:** Role-playing and skill-building exercises can help individuals develop social skills, such as active listening, empathy, and assertiveness, in a safe and supportive environment.

- **Encourage self-reflection:** Encouraging individuals to reflect on their social behaviors and the behaviors of others can help them develop self-awareness and promote the development of social skills. Developing social skills is an essential strategy for promoting social health. Encouraging participation in social activities, practicing active listening, offering positive reinforcement, role-playing and skill-building exercises, and encouraging self-reflection are all essential elements that can contribute to developing social skills and help individuals build meaningful relationships.

## Holistic Health Interventions

Mind-body interventions focus on the connection between the mind and the body and aim to promote overall health and wellness by addressing various physical, emotional, and spiritual aspects of a person's life. Social factors, such as relationships, social support, and community involvement, can significantly impact an individual's health and wellness and play an essential role in mind-body interventions.

For example, social support can provide individuals with the emotional and practical support they need to make positive lifestyle changes, such as regular exercise, maintaining a healthy diet, and managing stress. Community involvement can give individuals a sense of belonging, connection, and purpose, positively impacting their mental and emotional well-being.

Social aspects can be incorporated into specific mind-body interventions, such as yoga and meditation, which often encourage social connections and provide a sense of community among participants. For example, some yoga classes may incorporate partner poses or group

activities that promote social interaction and connection.

Overall, social aspects can play an essential role in various holistic health interventions, particularly mind-body interventions, by providing individuals with the social support and connection they need to promote social health.

## Complementary and Alternative Medicine

Social aspects can be crucial in various holistic health interventions, including complementary and alternative medicine (CAM). CAM refers to diverse medical and healthcare practices, therapies, and products not typically considered part of conventional medicine. Social factors, such as relationships, social support, and community involvement, can significantly impact an individual's health and well-being and play an essential role in CAM interventions.

Social support can provide individuals with the emotional and practical support they need to make positive lifestyle changes, such as regular exercise, maintaining a healthy diet, and managing stress.

Social aspects can also be incorporated into specific CAM interventions, such as acupuncture and massage therapy, which often involve interpersonal connections and provide a sense of comfort, relaxation, and fellowship among practitioners and recipients.

## Exercise and Nutrition

Both exercise and nutrition are essential components of holistic health, and social factors can impact an individual's ability to engage in healthy behaviors and make positive changes.

Social support is one of the most significant factors in promoting exercise and healthy eating. A supportive network of friends, family, or even an online community can provide the encouragement and motivation needed to sustain changes to one's exercise or eating habits. Additionally, having an exercise or nutrition partner can provide accountability and keep individuals on track with their goals.

Incorporating social aspects into exercise and nutrition interventions can also increase their effectiveness. Group fitness classes or workout groups can foster community and connection, providing additional motivation and support. Nutritional interventions that are conducted in a group setting provide opportunities for individuals to share their experiences, ask questions, and support each other in making healthy food choices.

## Psychotherapy and Counseling

Psychotherapy and counseling are therapeutic interventions that aim to improve a person's mental health and well-being. The inclusion of social factors can provide additional support and resources that can impact an individual's recovery and continued progress.

For example, social support from family, friends, or other community members can provide individuals with encouragement, validation, and positive reinforcement during the psychotherapy or counseling process. Social support can also provide individuals with the practical assistance needed to implement the skills and strategies learned in therapy.

Group therapy is also an effective form of psychotherapy that incorporates social aspects.

Group therapy allows individuals to connect with others who share similar experiences or concerns and can provide a sense of belonging and validation. Group therapy can also allow individuals to practice social skills and receive feedback in a safe and supportive environment.

Finally, culturally sensitive psychotherapy and counseling can consider the social and cultural factors that may impact a person's mental health and well-being. Taking these factors into account can help address underlying issues contributing to the individual's presenting symptoms.

## The Significance of Social Aspects

The significance of social aspects in holistic health cannot be overstated. The social determinants of health can have a powerful impact on our physical and emotional well-being, and addressing these determinants is essential for achieving better health outcomes.

At the individual level, social support networks have been shown to play a vital role in promoting resilience and reducing the impact of stressors on our health. Social support can also improve our ability to manage chronic diseases, speed up recovery times, and reduce the risk of hospitalization.

On a broader level, social determinants such as income, education, and access to healthcare can majorly impact overall health outcomes. Improving access to these resources can help reduce health disparities and promote health equity, ensuring that everyone has the opportunity to achieve their full potential for health and well-being.

## 5 More Minutes original author unknown

On a brisk autumn day, a lucky father took some time from his busy schedule to take his young daughter to the park near their house.

They reached the park, and the girl started playing on the toy bike in the playground. The father sat on a bench nearby and watched his daughter enjoy the beautiful day. After a while, a young woman sat down beside him. The woman beside him smiled and said, "That's my son over there." She pointed to a little boy in a blue sweater gliding down the slide. "He's a handsome boy," the man said. "That's my daughter on the bike in the pink dress."

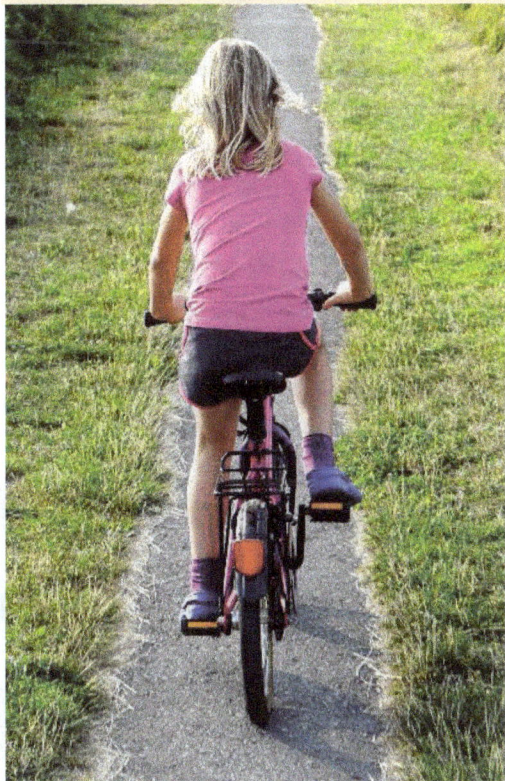

Then, looking at his watch, he called to his daughter. "What do you say, shall we go now?" His daughter pleaded, "No, just five more minutes, Dad. Please? Just five more minutes." The father nodded, and his daughter continued to ride the bike to her heart's content. Fifteen minutes passed, and he called again to his daughter. "Come on, it's time to go now." Once again the daughter pleaded, "Five more minutes, Dad.... give me just five more minutes." The father smiled and said, "Okay, Sweetheart." The girl continued playing. She was having fun, and his eyes were filled with happiness.

After 15 minutes or so, the same thing was repeated. He called to her, and she pleaded to allow her to play for a few more minutes and he happily permitted her to play for some more time.

The woman sitting next to him observed all this and was entirely surprised by the father's response. She said, "You certainly are a patient father. I appreciate your efforts to entertain your daughter's request again and again with a smiling face. If I had been in your place, I would have gotten annoyed."

The man smiled and replied, "Her older brother was killed while riding his bike and coming back home. I never spent much time with him and now I would give anything to spend just five more minutes with him. I've vowed not to make the same mistake with my daughter. She thinks she has five more minutes to ride the bike. The truth is, I get five more minutes to watch her play."

A great message conveyed through this story is to learn from your past mistakes. Accept them and ensure that you do not repeat them in the future. "Life can only be understood backward, but it must be lived forwards."

The story also conveys the importance of living in the present moment. The father understood the importance of the present moment. He not only noticed happiness after getting five more minutes, but he also had a self-awareness that he was giving five more minutes to himself to watch his daughter play.

In today's competitive environment, it seems that everyone prioritizes career and work. People have hectic routines to achieve their goals in their professional lives but need to maintain a good work-life balance. Spend some time with your family members and friends. In the story, the father in the story learned the hard way to prioritize his family above all others. No matter how busy things get, don't forget to spend time with people that matter to you!

Life is a race; it's all about making priorities. Do you have five more minutes? Give someone you love five more minutes today and see the difference, no matter how busy you are. You will have no regrets forever.

## Key Takeaways

The social aspect of health focuses on building and maintaining positive relationships with others. Social wellness includes developing and maintaining healthy relationships with family, friends, and colleagues and being part of a supportive community. Additionally, social wellness involves developing skills such as good communication, empathy, and active listening, which can help build solid relationships and connections with others. Overall, social wellness is an essential part of holistic health, and it is linked to improved mental and physical health, reduced stress, and a greater sense of well-being.

## Questions For Reflection:

1. Do I have a work-life balance?
2. If not, what can I do to achieve a work-life balance?
3. What can I add to my daily routine to socialize healthily?

## Take a Moment

_____
_____
_____
_____
_____
_____
_____
_____
_____
_____
_____
_____
_____
_____
_____
_____
_____
_____
_____
_____
_____
_____
_____
_____
_____
_____
_____
_____
_____
_____

In the next chapter, we will continue our learning journey and go into the spiritual aspects of holistic health, ways to nurture your spiritual health, and the importance of including a daily spiritual practice.

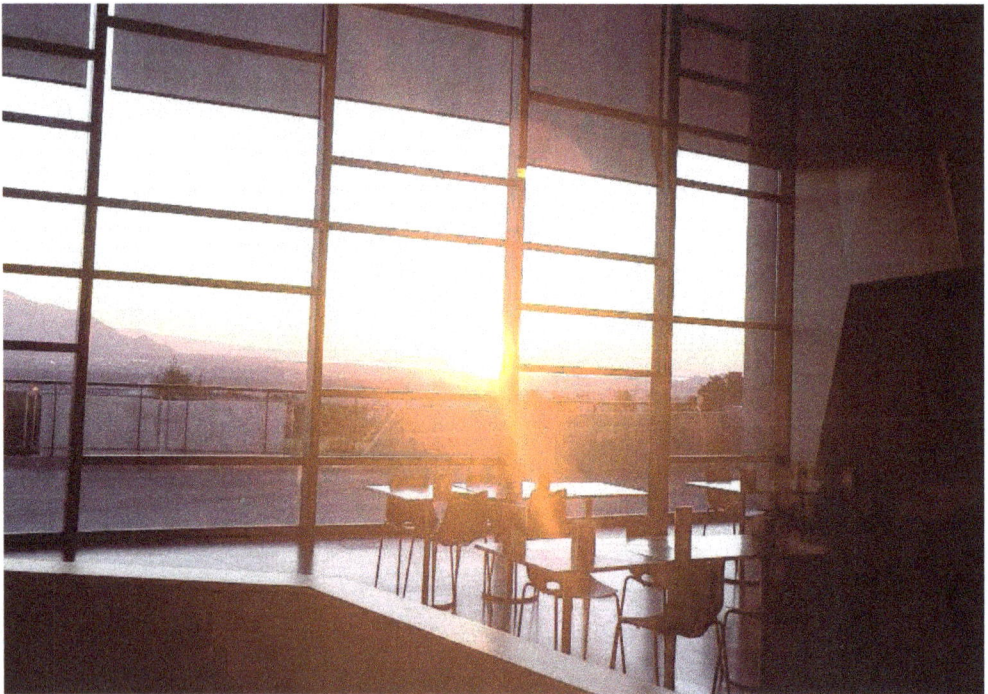

Image by Liesl Seborg

to have lower levels of stress and inflammation, which are risk factors for many chronic diseases.

Moreover, spirituality can also promote emotional health by helping individuals cope with stress, depression, and anxiety. By cultivating a sense of connection to a higher power or meaning in life, individuals can better cope with life's challenges and maintain a sense of optimism and hope.

Spirituality can play an essential role in supporting holistic health and well-being. By recognizing and addressing the spiritual dimension of health, individuals can achieve a sense of balance and harmony.

## Benefits of Nurturing Spiritualty

Nurturing spirituality can benefit individuals seeking to maintain or improve their holistic health. These benefits include improved mood, lower stress levels, better immune function, and improved sleep. Cultivating spirituality can also provide individuals with a greater sense of inner peace, strength, and purpose in life.

Nurturing spirituality in the context of holistic health can have several benefits, including:

- Promoting a sense of purpose and meaning
  Cultivating a sense of spirituality can help individuals connect with a purpose or meaning beyond themselves.
- Managing stress and anxiety
  Spirituality may help individuals cope with stress and anxiety by providing a sense of grounding, connectedness, and perspective.
- Promoting positive emotions
  Research has shown that spirituality is associated with enhanced positive emotions such as joy, gratitude, and compassion.

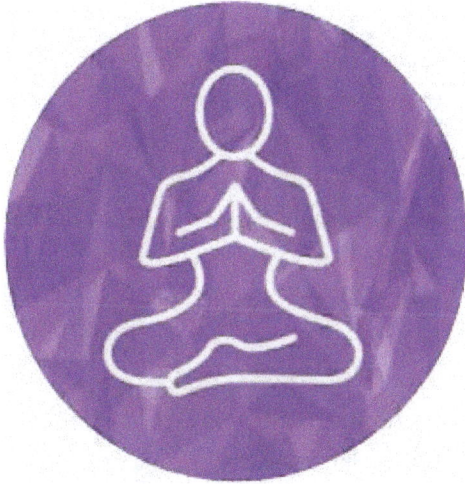

# Chapter Six: Spiritual Aspects of Holistic Health

*"What drains your spirit drains your body. What fuels your spirit fuels your body."*
*-Caroline Myss*

## The Importance of Spirituality

Spirituality is often defined as a connection to something greater than oneself, such as a higher power, purpose, or meaning. In holistic health, spirituality can provide a sense of purpose, meaning, and fulfillment that supports well-being.

Research has shown that spirituality can positively impact physical health by promoting healthy behaviors and reducing the risk of chronic conditions such as heart disease and cancer. For example, individuals who practice regular meditation or prayer have been shown

- Supporting physical health
  Some studies suggest that spirituality positively impacts physical health by reducing inflammation, promoting healthy behaviors, and improving immune function.
- Deepening personal relationships
  Spirituality can sometimes foster more profound and meaningful connections with others as individuals connect around shared beliefs or ideals.

The spiritual aspect of holistic health often needs to be addressed alongside social health. Nurturing one's spirituality can contribute to overall wellness by promoting emotional, relational, and physical health. So, let's not just focus on the physical and mental side of holistic health. Let's focus on all areas of holistic health, including the spiritual.

## Factors Affecting Spiritual Health

Some of the factors affecting spiritual health include:

- Academic or employment stress
- Life dissatisfaction
- Religious problems or questioning of faith
- Culture and gender
- Personal beliefs and values
- External factors, such as societal and environmental factors
- The individual's sense of purpose and meaning in life
- Spirituality and religiosity
- Mental health and well-being
- Social support and relationships

Various factors can impact an individual's spiritual health, and these factors vary based on individual experiences, cultural and societal backgrounds, and personal beliefs and values. Understanding the factors contributing to spiritual health can help individuals integrate spirituality into their healthcare practices.

## SPIRITUAL HEALTH FIRST STEPS

- PRACTICE MEDITATION OR PRAYER
- SPEND TIME IN NATURE
- ENGAGE IN ACTS OF SERVICE
- CULTIVATE GRATITUDE
- SEEK OUT MEANINGFUL CONNECTIONS

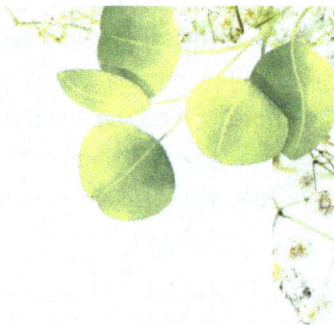

## Spiritual Experience by Sharry

I had a repetitive injury that "necessitated a surgical repair," so the doctors said. This was a work-related injury, and workman's compensation would cover the surgery and follow-up care, but only if I followed the doctor's instructions. I needed the job, so I had the surgery and followed the doctor's and physical therapist's instructions, but I was not healing. My shoulder became stiff and left me with limited use of my right arm. I was tired, hurting badly all the time, and my blood pressure was elevated, but no one knew why. I was declared disabled and left to my own devices. This went on for 12 years until I found an answer from God.

Years earlier, I had heard from God and began to listen to the voice. My life changed a lot, leaving an abusive boyfriend, letting go of bad habits, and seeing life and other people as blessings. I felt His forgiveness for my previous bad behavior and lifestyle.

As a child, I was taught that God was some fierce entity at the end of the universe who was unreachable, sat in judgment, and couldn't wait to condemn me to hell the next time I took a pencil from the bank by mistake. I left the church I which I was raised and paid no mind to religion. But when He came and called me, I learned that He is the good guy and He's on my side. I remember the day. I was getting ready for work that morning, putting on my makeup and doing my hair, and I heard a voice say, "God." Soft and quiet, yet it got my attention.

I began a search for God in religions, cultures, and philosophies. There are so many different beliefs that all claim to be the right way. Just as I was starting my search, my injury and subsequent surgery occurred. Since I couldn't work and spent lots of time in bed coping with the pain, I had lots of time to read. I learned so much about how God can come to us where we are and guide us along His chosen path, but we must be quiet and listen.

I learned that He uses these situations to teach us something we will need later in life. I realized that I wasn't being punished, but the pain, weakness, and dismissal by doctors and other people were grooming me for a purpose to come. And it came.

God sent me an angel at the end of the 12 years, which I now see as a precious time—a physical therapist who had a different approach to my stiff and painful shoulder. On the first visit, something lit up inside me the minute he put his hands on my back. It's something that cannot be named or described. It felt so real, so natural, and it worked. Myofascial Release, as taught by John Barnes, was the type of bodywork he performed. Over a few months, my body began to heal. My shoulder loosened, the pain decreased significantly, and I felt more alive.

One day, during a treatment, God came into the room. It was a light that I had never seen before or since. It was interesting, as the window shades were closed, and a small lamp was in the room. And here came the voice again. It said, "Learn to share this blessing. I will lift you." So I did. I learned to share the blessing, and God lifted me physically, financially, and socially. Every aspect of my life has been improved. And I owe it all to God.

## Life Creed by Sharry

Life is no accident. Everyone and everything has been created on purpose, for a purpose, by One Much Higher than ourselves.

We must respect this gift of life, see the good in others, and reach out and help those we can, for we are all one.

The Africans teach word sound power. Everything we say - every syllable, every utterance - comes from a vibration that begins in the thought, travels through the throat and out the mouth, and circles the globe as it leaves the body. It will affect someone somewhere in the world. We must ensure that the things we say are positive to have a positive effect. All things, good and bad, are necessary to balance the circle of life.

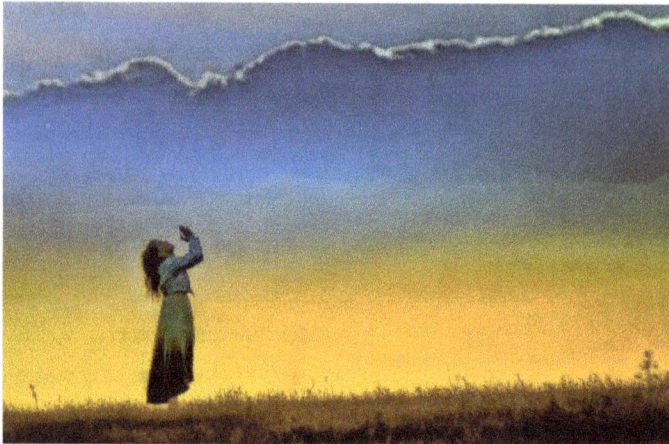

There are evils on the earth, and they do serve their purpose. But, I serve a positive purpose, bring a positive vibration, and serve a Higher Power. And I do it in His Name.

One love. October 26, 2013.

## Spiritual Support Networks

Several organizations provide spiritual support networks for patients and their families. Some of these networks are part of spiritual care services offered by hospitals and healthcare facilities, while others are independent organizations that bring together healthcare professionals and spiritual leaders.

Examples of spiritual support networks include:

- The Spiritual Care Network
- Spiritual Support Services at GBMC HealthCare
- Visualizing Spiritual Support Networks
- Services at healthcare facilities
- Pastoral care services and prayer groups offered by chaplains and spiritual leaders

Spiritual support networks can provide emotional and spiritual support to individuals and families navigating health challenges. These networks offer community and connection and help individuals and families build resilience during difficult times.

## Spiritual Resources

Spiritual resources are available through various avenues, including healthcare facilities, religious organizations, and online resources.

These resources can include campus ministry programs, chaplaincy departments, prayer groups, and spiritual counseling services. Many online resources are also available, that include spiritual reading materials, daily prayer resources, and virtual worship services.

While access to spiritual resources may vary depending on an individual's location and circumstances, many resources are available to those seeking spiritual support and connection. Clients and their families can work with holistic health providers to identify and access spiritual resources during times of illness or crisis, and individuals can also seek out help and support through their local religious communities or online.

## Native American and Ancient Healing by Stephanie

The word "healing" is used in many ways, but to Native Americans, it is more than just fending off invading disease, it also refers to the body regenerating itself after injury or illness. Healing considers that our bodies are not separate from our thoughts, emotions, or souls. For this reason, healing takes on a deeper meaning in Native American traditions and Ancient healing practices.

Many people are unaware of the connection between the onset of illness and the underlying energetic changes in their body and don't realize that their state of mind, or outlook on life, affects their physical health as much, if not more, than what they eat or how much they sleep. The body keeps its systems balanced to fight off invaders that permit illness to take hold. Changes on the cellular level brought on by negative mental or emotional states, such as sadness, grief, anger, resentment, hate, regret, shame, loneliness, or stress, can weaken our immune systems and even turn our cells against us.

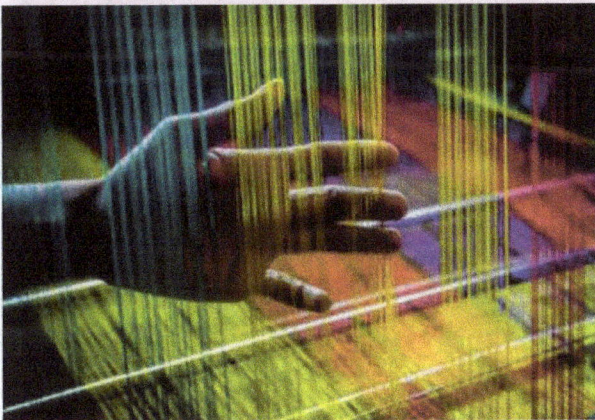

We can change how we view healing and weave back restoration, like a great tapestry torn by time and trauma that has been stained or abused. It takes more than simple repairs or closing up of holes to return to its original beauty. When the body is weak or sick, more is needed than chemical remedies to kill germs or fool unbalanced systems. Rebalancing and reunifying all aspects of the Self are required to mend and reweave our energetic systems. This reunification must reconnect the shredded fibers of the body, mind, emotions, and soul. True healing is gaining balance of what we are, how we think, what we feel, what we do, and how we live on all levels of our lives simultaneously.

Native Americans believe that healing involves increasing our ability to accept life and let go of what has been in order to release our imbalanced state. This allows us to expand and grow as souls, for most often, it is resistance to change and the flow of life events that has brought on stress, imbalance, or weakness in the first place. This process is often invisible to us, but when we encounter a painful occurrence we can't cope with or understand physically, emotionally, mentally, or spiritually, we get hurt, become ill, or split off some of our spirit and consciousness, which weakens us. If we are willing to do the work to look honestly inside of ourselves, face whatever illness or trauma is there, learn from it, and allow healing change, we can reconnect to our spirit and consciousness. Through this process, we can evolve our souls and achieve "health."

Nearly all of us have unresolved physical, emotional, mental, or spiritual issues, some of which we are unaware of or in denial about. It is important to remember that everyone can benefit from the processes of healing as a way to resolve these issues and move to a higher awareness. True healing is an exploration of self-discovery and an opportunity for personal enlightenment that we can all benefit from. It takes courage to take on your healing, but by doing so, you will embark on a transformation process that will expand your mind, heart, and soul.

Native Americans believe that anything can be healed, including our ability to heal ourselves, but sometimes, we need more energy, understanding, or love than we can muster to achieve. These are the times when we must be willing to accept help from others, whether they are family, friends, or trained professionals skilled in the healing arts.

Each of us is made up of many elements on many levels. Some are dense and physical, while others are higher in vibration. Our minds and emotions are collections of swimming patterns of energy, feelings, thoughts, and consciousness that never stop. These identity fragments are connected with our physicality and rule over our bodily functions, yet they sometimes seem to exist in their private world. At the highest level, we are pure energy and spirit. Here, we see the parts of ourselves that are metaphysical, which go beyond the realm of matter and intertwine with other people, dimensions, and the Universal Consciousness or God. Of all these levels, it is through the mind that we have access to the most power, for through thought and consciousness, we can create or destroy the delicate balances that exist between us and the outside world.

What would it be like if you were whole? How would that change your reality if you knew who you are, where you came from, and what you are here to do? Tapping into these inner resources is what healing is all about. What would it be like to enjoy perfect, robust health and complete peace in your mind and emotions?  We are talking about regaining the elements of ourselves that have become shut down, split off, or suppressed to the point that we feel lost, weak, incapable, angry, depressed, powerless, or just plain sick. This fragmentation diffuses our energy and attention and causes us to be no longer able to fully engage in life the way we should or the way we dream of.

For many of us, this breaking apart of the Self may have started early in life or as long as we can remember, which have felt like chains that hold us back from our heart's desires. We are not separate from our minds, emotions, and spiritual bodies. Therefore, we must heal all aspects of ourselves while supporting, guiding, and even challenging ourselves as we walk toward recovery.

## Holistic Health Interventions

Spiritual aspects are recognized as a vital component of various holistic health interventions. Integrating spiritual care into conventional healthcare practices, including complementary, alternative, and integrative health interventions, can help address the spiritual dimension of well-being.

Studies suggest that incorporating spiritual practices, such as yoga and mindfulness meditation, into healthcare interventions can positively impact physical and mental health outcomes. Religious and spiritually based activities have also promoted mental, physical, and spiritual health.

Recognizing and addressing spiritual needs as a part of healthcare practices can improve client outcomes and promote well-being. This integration of spiritual aspects into holistic healthcare interventions can support individuals to achieve a state of optimal health.

## The Significance of Spiritual Aspects

Reflecting on the significance of spiritual aspects in holistic health, it is clear that spiritual health is essential to health and well-being. The spiritual dimension of health is considered by many to be the foundation of holistic health, which aims to treat the whole person, not just their physical symptoms.

Incorporating spiritual aspects into holistic health interventions also brings a sense of meaning and purpose to individuals' lives. Spiritual care is a critical component of patient-centered care, which is focused on tailoring care to meet each patient's individual needs, beliefs, and values.

By acknowledging and addressing the spiritual dimension of well-being, holistic health providers can offer more comprehensive and personalized care to supports individuals in achieving their health goals.

## Spirits Touching by Debbie Hillyard, Diet Assistant

I met a very elderly patient recently. She was very thin, malnourished, and had been found in a coma.

As we cared for her, she began to revive, although her speech was very slurred, and her mind vacillated from lucid to foggy. It took her a long time, with much help, to inform me about her food sensitivities.

At the end of our long conversation, she asked me my first and last names, then mumbled, "We are now forever friends. We know each other after a short visit and will now be friends for life!"

I immediately resonated with my patient and said, "Yes, we are indeed life friends!" I assured her I would check in again and conveyed how much I treasured her and her sweetness. She seemed very grateful when I added that I would be thinking of and praying for her.

This dear woman began failing the next day and never ate or spoke again. Reading her obituary the following week, I

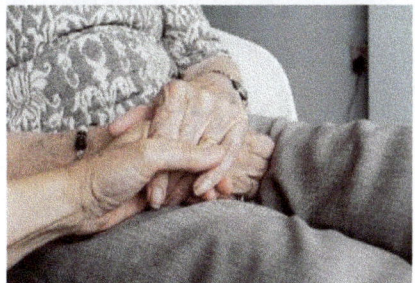

Image by Sabine van Erp

93

discovered that she had been a ministry leader for many decades and that her "mission in life was to share the love of Jesus." My most extraordinary mission is to "be God in the skin" to all I encounter.

So our spirits indeed had been in total resonance the day we spoke, even though we had just met. The depth of connection I shared with her remains imprinted in my heart, soul, and spirit, and I look forward to our future relationship in heavenly places.

I have experienced many of these types of soul and spiritual connections, often with dying people, and they always leave me touched and feeling blessed. The link never ceases and will continue even after we all graduate to a higher spirit realm.

## Key Takeaways

The spiritual dimension of wellness is an essential aspect of holistic health that involves finding meaning and purpose in life and developing a sense of inner peace and connection with something greater than oneself. The key takeaways regarding the spiritual aspect of holistic health are:

- Spiritual wellness is one of the five aspects of holistic health and is crucial to achieving a balanced and fulfilling life.
- Spiritual wellness involves finding meaning and purpose through self-reflection, meditation, prayer, or other spiritual practices.
- Developing a sense of inner peace and connection with something greater than oneself can help reduce stress, anxiety, and depression and improve mental health.
- Spirituality is not necessarily tied to religion and can involve a personal belief system or connection to nature or the universe.
- Integrating spirituality into everyday life can enhance the overall well-being of an individual by promoting a sense of balance, harmony, and purpose.
- Holistic health is an approach that recognizes that a person's physical, emotional, mental, and spiritual aspects are interconnected and influence each other. Therefore, spiritual wellness is an integral component of holistic health that cannot be ignored.

# Questions For Reflection:

1. Have I experienced a deep connection with a particular individual? What was it about that person that resonated with me?
2. What do these connections tell us about ourselves, the spirit, the presence of God/Creator/Universe/ Great Spirit in this world?

*Take a Moment*

_____
_____
_____
_____
_____
_____
_____
_____
_____
_____
_____
_____
_____
_____
_____
_____
_____
_____
_____

_____
_____
_____
_____
_____
_____
_____
_____
_____
_____
_____
_____
_____

In the next and final chapter, you will learn about the emotional aspects of holistic health, its benefits, importance, and ways to nurture emotional well-being with self-care and professional assistance.

Image by Stephanie Seborg

Emotionally healthy individuals can cope with stress, have stronger relationships, and are better equipped to handle life's challenges. On the other hand, poor emotional health can lead to a range of adverse outcomes, including poor physical health, mental health issues, and reduced quality of life.

Therefore, addressing emotional health should be a core aspect of any holistic health approach. It is essential to focus on improving emotional well-being and empowering individuals to better manage their feelings and emotions in a way that supports their overall health and well-being.

Emotional health is intimately linked to physical and mental health, and poor emotional health can lead to various adverse outcomes, including chronic stress, anxiety, depression, and physical illnesses. On the other hand, good emotional health can lead to enhanced coping skills, resilience, and improved emotional regulation.

## Benefits of Nurturing Emotional Health

Nurturing emotional health can have many benefits for individuals seeking to maintain or improve their holistic health. These benefits include increased resilience, improved coping skills, enhanced relationships, better decision-making skills, and overall well-being. Cultivating emotional health can also lead to more significant social connections, increased motivation, and better physical health.

Nurturing emotional health is an essential aspect of holistic health, as it has been linked to various benefits. Some of these benefits include:

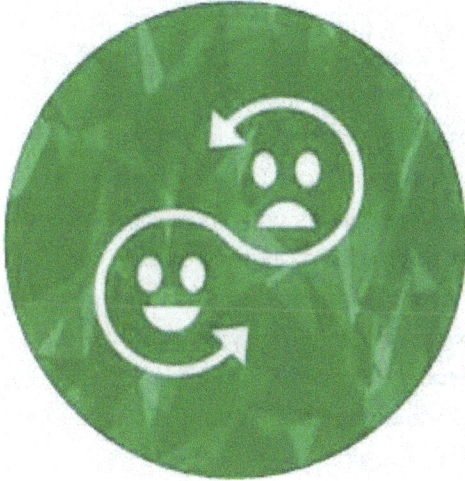

# Chapter Seven: Emotional Aspects of Holistic Health

*"Happiness is the highest form of health."*
*-Dalai Lama*

## The Importance of Emotional Health in Holistic Health

Emotional health is a critical component of holistic health. It refers to an individual's ability to manage, understand, and express their emotions healthily and positively. Emotional health is essential to well-being and is linked to physical health, mental health, and social functioning.

- Improved mental health: Nurturing emotional health can reduce the risk of developing mental disorders such as depression, anxiety, and stress.
- Better physical health: Emotional health is closely linked to physical health; improving emotional well-being can lead to improved physical health outcomes.
- Increased resilience: Emotionally healthy individuals are better able to cope with the challenges of daily life, including stress, grief, and loss.
- Stronger relationships: Nurturing emotional health can lead to better communication skills, improved empathy, and stronger interpersonal relationships.
- Improved quality of life: Emotional health is an essential aspect of overall well-being and nurturing emotional health can lead to increased happiness, contentment, and fulfillment in life.

Being confronted with a health issue can bring out strong emotions. Pain, fever, weakness, digestive troubles, and other symptoms are some of the things that can change our emotional state. How others treat and speak to you can also influence your emotions. Just because you cannot do the things you used to or want to do can lead to some powerful and heavy feelings.

## They Simply Don't Know by Sharry

When I was dealing with being "disabled," I began to journal, then decided to write a book about how our lives change when we become "disabled." I put that word into quotes because I learned that if I keep thinking of myself that way, I will not be able to heal or recover. I thought of myself as "lesser-abled."

And, by the way, I did heal, which is why I felt called to help others heal as well.

When we get injured or seriously ill in a way that takes a few months or even a few years for us to heal, our minds are affected, as well as our bodies. We are unable to move as we did before. Working, shopping, and enjoying a hobby can be aggravating, frustrating, and depressing. These emotions are common side effects of long-term recovery.

Most of us have had a bad cold or the flu that kept us home in bed for several days or more. But, to be held at home or in bed for six months, nine months, or a couple of years is very difficult to deal with. We think, "A couple more weeks (or months) and I'll be okay." After two years of "two more weeks," one can almost give up on ever being well again. Relief becomes a goal that we seek but never attain. Add that to discussing the pain and suffering, often reinforced by people who think they are helping. Bless their hearts; we know they mean well. But just the opposite is true. Asking how we feel, offering suggestions, and feeling sorry for us only makes it worse.

I learned to give thanks for and appreciate the things I could do. I could bathe and dress myself, drive myself to the store and doctors' visits. I had income to pay the bills, and was getting by okay.

I realized that getting well would have to start with how I saw myself. Now that I had accepted my disability and had made the necessary adjustments, I was ready to move on.

I began to joke with myself about my gimp. "Gimp" is the term I used to describe the injuries and arthritis that I dealt with. It's a general term, and it's a term that made me laugh. We can either laugh or cry about our disabilities, and laughing is a lot more fun. Some people will tell us, "You shouldn't think of yourself that way." These people don't understand that we are lifting our spirits and finding enjoyment in life by doing this. Laughter can cause our depression to ease up and can decrease our pain.

I remember talking with a woman who asked the famous question, "How are you feeling?"

"I'm doing well," I replied, "Thanks."

"Oh? So you don't hurt anymore?"

"Oh, no, it still hurts like hell."

"Well, then, how can you say you're okay?" she asked in an agitated voice, then she turned and walked away.

I said nothing but thought to myself, "Excuse me for looking on the bright side."

When others see us dealing with lesser abilities, they become afraid of us, not because of who we are, but because they see themselves as possibly having to deal with this at some point. No one sees this coming. It is a shock and a disappointment when one becomes disabled and ill for an extended period or even a lifetime. An average healthy person doesn't think about this until they see someone limping or struggling. These things happen to someone else. But it's a whole different story when that someone else is you.

No one but ourselves knows how we feel inside. Physically, the pain and weakness that we deal with can affect our lives dramatically. Little everyday tasks are slow, complex, or even impossible. Emotionally, the hurt and aggravation of needing help to get through the day can be

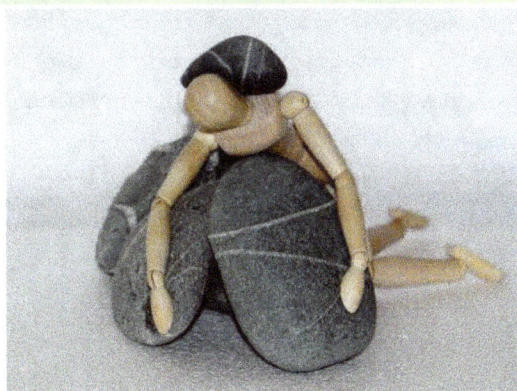
Image by Counseling

overwhelming. After several months go by, depression likes to move in. We can become isolated as our friends, family, and neighbors go about their lives. Wish as we might, we cannot do things like we once did, and it takes time and conscious effort to accept this.

We liken our slow, painful movements to those of older folks. I think we relate to living like older folks because it's the closest example we have to follow. A person with a healthy body cannot understand how we feel. One must experience it personally to know how it is to live slowly and painfully.

I realized that while living like an older person, my thinking was also slowing. The world suddenly was moving too fast! At the grocery store checkout, the cashier was scanning my items at lightning speed (or so it seemed to me), and I tried very hard, with my fuzzy mind, to comprehend the money she was asking me to pay. Going to the store was a regular activity for me six months ago. Why did it seem so foreign to me now?

I recall we had attended an event: my son, his friend, and myself. All went well until we were in the parking lot, walking to the car to leave. The kids didn't realize how slow I had to walk (me and my cane). I remember standing in the middle of a crowd of people, cars and headlights coming from all directions, horns honking, folks pushing past me. I looked ahead to see if I could see the kids or the car and noticed my son's friend briskly walking way out ahead and my son about halfway between us, looking at me very uncertainly. The friend noticed that her companions were lagging. Too far ahead to hear my son shout, "We have to wait for Mom." I was so scared and felt so helpless and alone. I felt embarrassed that I had let them down. After all, this was the mom who would have raced them to the car a year earlier.

I've never told anyone this because I don't want to make anyone feel bad. They didn't know. But that moment is still very vivid in my mind even though it was nine years ago at this writing.

It's been said that living with and being around younger folks will keep you young. This is true to a degree. But it can also remind you of what you used to do but now can't. I remember speaking with one young person about exercise and how I'm doing pretty well but still not quite there. This young person suggested that I could get over it if I worked harder. This is lovely advice for a healthy person wanting to get stronger, but very dangerous for someone with already damaged muscles and joints.

Folks in the medical field, the doctors and nurses that we see regularly, do an excellent job with the knowledge and skills that they have. However, I would like to explain to them that we do not want to be referred to as patients, sufferers, victims, or 'people your age.' Hearing these terms does not lead to a positive self-view. Psychology has taught us that what we hear, think, and say about ourselves we begin to believe. This is called environmental conditioning. So, when I heard myself being called an older person, I began to feel and act older. At first, I had to accept it, acceptance of being part of the situation. However, as I began to take control of my healing and had no more weekly doctor visits, I began to feel younger.

I read an article in a popular magazine about a woman dealing with cancer who hated being seen as a "sick" person or a "patient." She wrote that her life had become centered on cancer and that she hadn't felt the urge to start checking off wishes on a life list. While arthritis is not life-threatening, I can relate to this woman; her life is about cancer, and my life is about arthritis.

I know now that moving my mind away from those terms greatly affected my recovery. Perhaps we should ask our medical professionals not to use these terms with us but rather to refer to us as simply "a man, woman, or person dealing with a situation."

They don't mean to offend anyone. I worked in a nursing home early in my career and was probably guilty of sounding like that myself. But I didn't know. I treated people like the older nurses, and aides did; it was part of the training.

There was another article in a popular magazine by a man writing about his experiences while paralyzed from an accident. He talked about the nurses and aids who came into his hospital room with their 'sing-song chirpy-chirpy, how are we today' nonsense. I have heard those voices, and now I see how ridiculous it sounds.

Lesser-abled people don't get that kind of treatment from everyone, but it can happen enough times to make it unpleasant to go out in public sometimes. I would often stay home if I were not in the mood to hear the advice and sympathy. And when I encounter the 'helper,' I try to shrug it off with humor or change the subject. I feel it's essential always to behave your best, even when dealing with someone who is "just trying to help." I say, "Thank you. I love you, but I don't need help."

It only takes a couple of times for hurt to set in after someone has given a look or commented about how we do things. Since we spend so much time alone, our thoughts can often drift to remembering these situations, and we can dwell on them too long. This can exaggerate the problem and make it seem like it happens more than it does. We have to get out and socialize to keep ourselves mentally fit. We must learn to deal with these helpful people and still show them respect, even if we don't get it ourselves.

Developing and keeping a positive attitude is challenging when others constantly want to point out the situation. We are aware of our situation. And we want to live our lives without all the discussion.

I hope this little story helps you in some way.

## Holistic Emotional Health

In practice, emotional health is an essential component of holistic health and many therapeutic approaches and self-care methods focus on addressing emotional health. For example, Cognitive Behavioral Therapy (CBT) and Dialectical Behavioral Therapy (DBT) focus on regulating emotions and developing healthy coping skills. Holistic emotional health emphasizes the importance of self-care, self-awareness, and self-reflection in maintaining health. It involves practices and strategies that promote emotional well-being and help individuals cope with life's challenges. Practices for holistic emotional health are:

- Self-care: Self-care is about engaging in activities that promote health.
- Emotional Awareness: Emotional awareness involves recognizing and coming to an understanding of one's emotions.
- Stress Management: Learning techniques to manage stress may include deep breathing exercises, practicing mindfulness, engaging in stress-reducing activities, and setting personal boundaries.

- Healthy Relationships: It is vital to foster positive connections with friends, family, and other supportive individuals.

EMOTIONAL HEALTH
FIRST STEPS

- SURROUND YOURSELF WITH SUPPORTIVE PEOPLE
- LOOK INWARD FOR VALIDATION
- REGULARLY EXERCISE AND EAT HEALTHY MEALS
- PRACTICE SELF-CARE
- TRY NEW THINGS
- SEEK SUPPORT WHEN NEEDED

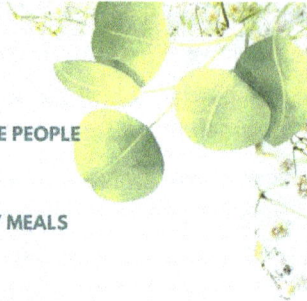

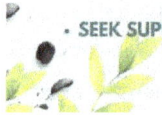

## Factors Affecting Emotional Health

Here are some factors that can affect emotional health:

- Life events: Changes in work, school, relationships, or home life, as well as significant life events such as becoming a parent, can impact emotional health.
- Environmental factors: The environment in which a person lives can impact emotional health, including exposure to toxins, access to green spaces, and exposure to noise pollution.
- Genetics: Genetics can play a role in emotional health, with certain genetic factors increasing the risk for mental health disorders.
- Stress: Experiencing chronic or acute stress can impact emotional health, increasing the risk for mental health disorders such as anxiety and depression.
- Diet and nutrition: Poor nutrition can negatively impact emotional health, contributing to mood disorders and other mental health conditions.
- Physical inactivity: Lack of exercise and physical activity has been linked to poorer emotional health outcomes.
- Social support: A lack of social support, isolation, and loneliness can impact emotional health, increasing the risk for depression and other mental health issues.

Overall, emotional health is influenced by various factors, including life events, environmental factors, genetics, stress, diet and nutrition, physical inactivity, and social support.

## Emotional Support Networks

Emotional support networks refer to a group of trusted individuals to turn to for support during difficult times. These networks are typically made up of friends, family members, and colleagues who offer emotional support, empathy, and understanding.

Emotional support networks are essential in maintaining mental health and well-being, providing individuals with a sense of belonging, connectedness, and social support. Studies have shown that having a strong emotional support network can help reduce the risk of depression and anxiety, improve coping skills during stressful situations, and promote overall psychological well-being. Dynamic support networks can be built and strengthened through regular social interactions, open communication, and mutual support.

Additionally, seeking professional help from mental health professionals such as therapists and counselors can be an essential part of an individual's emotional support network.

## Access to Emotional Health Resources

There are many options for accessing emotional health resources:

- VA Mental Health Services: Veterans can access mental health services through the VA for conditions such as PTSD and military sexual trauma.
- Mental Health Services: There are a variety of mental health services available to the general public, including crisis lines, consumer-operated warm lines, and behavioral health services. Many providers offer 24/7 support.
- SAMHSA: The Substance Abuse and Mental Health Services Administration is an excellent resource for information on mental health and to locate treatment services in your area.
- Children's Mental Health Care: The CDC is committed to helping children and families get the mental health care they need and

provide resources and information on improving access to care.
- Aetna Mental Health & Well-being Resources: Aetna, a CVS Health company, offers resources to support the whole person, including emotional health. They also have member access to quality behavioral and mental health resources.
- Kaiser Permanente Mental Health & Wellness: Kaiser Permanente offers its members comprehensive, integrated mental health care, including access to services under their Medicaid plan.

Emotional health resources are numerous. People can access mental health services through the VA, crisis hotlines, SAMSHA, and other resources. Additionally, many insurance plans offer mental health coverage and telehealth services, making receiving care from the comfort of your home more accessible. At the end of this book, you will find a resource section listing the different mental health services listed above.

## Emotional Aspects in Interventions

Various holistic health interventions acknowledge the importance of emotional aspects. Emotional health is considered an integral component of overall well-being in holism. Below are some examples of how emotional elements are incorporated into different holistic health interventions:

- Mindfulness-based interventions: Mindfulness practices focus on developing non-judgmental awareness and acceptance of the present moment, including one's thoughts, emotions, and physical sensations.

- **Holistic healthcare interventions for children:** Emotional and mental health are included in the biopsychosocial model of holistic healthcare, emphasizing that all aspects of a child's life are interconnected.
- **Disaster management and its impact on mental health:** Natural disasters can have significant emotional and psychological effects on individuals, and appropriate support and interventions must be implemented to address these impacts.
- **The PERMA model of happiness:** The PERMA model is a framework for measuring and promoting well-being, which includes positive emotions as one of its key components.
  https://positivepsychology.com/perma-model/
- **Spirituality and health:** Spirituality has been linked to improved emotional and mental health, and many holistic healthcare interventions emphasize the importance of spiritual well-being.

Holistic healthcare interventions recognize the importance of emotional aspects in overall well-being, and many interventions incorporate emotional health as a critical component. Mindfulness practices, the biopsychosocial model, disaster management, the PERMA model, and spirituality are examples of how emotional aspects are incorporated into different holistic health interventions.

## Significance of Emotional Aspects

Emotional aspects are crucial in holistic health as they significantly impact an individual's well-being. Holistic health recognizes that the mind, body, and spirit are interconnected and that an individual's emotions and feelings play a vital role in their health. Negative emotions, such as stress, anxiety, depression, and fear, can harm physical and mental health, leading to a range of health issues.

Moreover, emotional aspects are essential components of holistic health interventions. Mindfulness practices, spirituality, and positive psychology-based interventions encourage individuals to recognize, explore, and manage their emotions effectively for improved overall well-being. For instance, meditation and mindfulness cultivate awareness and acceptance of emotions, which helps individuals cope with stress and manage their emotional responses more effectively.

Emotional support and compassion are integral parts of holistic healthcare interventions. A holistic approach to healthcare addresses the spiritual, emotional, and social aspects of a patient's life. It recognizes the significance of positive relationships and social connections in promoting overall well-being.

In conclusion, emotions and feelings play an essential role in holistic health, and addressing them is fundamental to achieving optimal physical, mental, and spiritual well-being. By recognizing and addressing the emotional aspects of an individual's life, holistic health interventions offer a more comprehensive approach to healthcare that supports overall wellness and improved quality of life.

## Happiness is Within You adapted from the Persian Folktale

Once there was a wealthy man who lived in abundance in a castle on the hill. He had no want or need but he was always worried and restless. One day while touring the countryside, he met a sage at the edge of the forest. The wealthy man shared his problem with the sage, that he had no shortage of anything yet always worried and was unhappy.

The sage heard his problem and replied calmly, "Come tomorrow, and I will tell you how to stay happy and worry-free."

The next day, the man went to the edge of the forest and saw the sage was looking for something outside his humble hut.

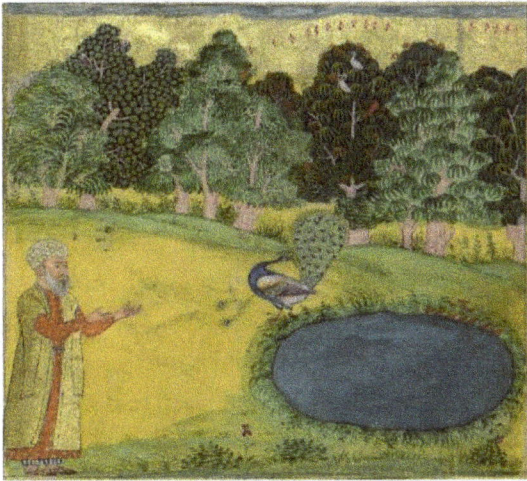

The man asked, "What are you looking for? May I help you?"

The sage replied, "I have lost my ring and am searching for it."

After hearing this, the man began searching for the ring alongside the sage. After searching for nearly an hour, the ring was not found. The wealthy man then asked the sage, "Where did your ring fall exactly?"

The sage said, "My ring fell in my humble hut. But it is very dark there, so I am looking for the ring outside."

Surprised, the man asked, "If your ring fell in your hut, then why are you looking out here??? How will you find the thing outside, which is inside there?"

The sage smiled and replied, "My dear son, this is the solution to your problem."

The man looked at the sage with curious eyes. The sage continued, "You came with the problem that you have no shortage of anything, but you are still unhappy with your life. Happiness is right there inside you, but you are looking for it outside in the materialistic world."

The sage added, smiling, "The entire ocean is inside you, but still, you are looking for water outside with a spoon. Money or property is important, but happiness cannot be bought with money. Look for the happiness within you; it's there, and you do not need to search for it in the outside world."

We often search outside ourselves for the happiness that has been inside all along. Instead of telling the person the secret of joy during his first visit, the sage explained it the next day with an example. The sage taught him the lesson of connecting with an incident, which is always more valuable. The source of happiness is within us. Happiness starts from within us.

Happiness is often the result of external factors, but the natural source of happiness comes from within you. There is inner happiness within everyone, but layers of negative thoughts, fears, worries, and anxieties cover it. Inner happiness is an inseparable part of our inner being and essence. But we often allow various factors to hide it.

Happiness, in truth, lies within you. It starts with you and ends with you. Happiness and peace are two primary characteristics of every soul. You do not have to chase it, climb a thousand stairs, or learn rocket science to experience it.

Many people try to look for happiness through their wealth, career, money, and success. They feel surprised not to experience happiness even when having a penthouse apartment overlooking the London Eye next to the Houses of Parliament and earning seven figures annually. Happiness is something we choose for ourselves and how we choose to live our lives according to our being. It is not following someone else's rhythm as it is our own. It is our inner feeling that creates happiness, along with how we interpret the events of life.

## Key Takeaways

The emotional aspects of holistic health are essential for overall well-being because they impact mental health, improve coping skills, and promote healthy behaviors. Here are some key takeaways:

- Emotional wellness is one of the dimensions of holistic health and involves being aware of and accepting one's feelings, managing emotions effectively, and coping with stress.
- Emotional wellness contributes to overall well-being by improving mental health, promoting healthy behaviors, enhancing relationships, and increasing resilience.
- Emotions impact physical health, so nurturing emotional wellness can help reduce the risk of chronic diseases and other physical health problems.
- Emotional wellness is vital to managing stress, significantly contributing to poor mental and physical health.
- Strategies for cultivating emotional wellness include mindfulness practices, expressing emotions, seeking needed support, and engaging in activities that bring joy and fulfillment.

Overall, emotional wellness is an essential part of holistic health. It impacts mental health, improves coping skills, and promotes healthy behaviors, making it crucial for achieving overall well-being.

# Questions For Reflection:

1. **Do I feel my emotional health could be better or improved?**
2. **What are some holistic ways to support and nurture my emotional health?**

*Take a Moment*

_____
_____
_____
_____
_____
_____
_____
_____
_____
_____
_____
_____
_____
_____
_____
_____
_____
_____
_____
_____

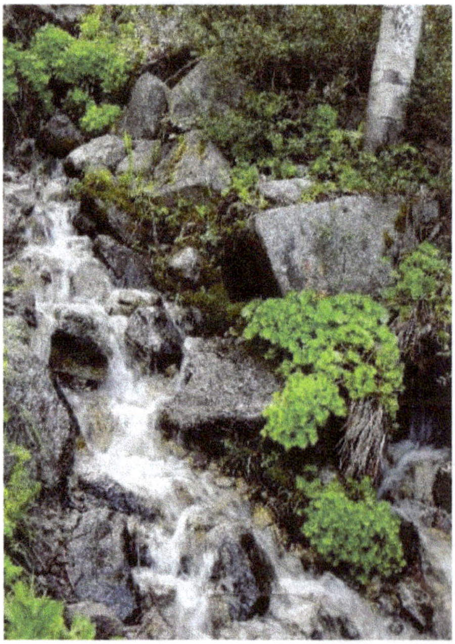

_____
_____
_____
_____
_____
_____
_____
_____
_____
_____
_____
_____
_____
_____
_____
_____
_____
_____
_____

Image by Stephanie Seborg

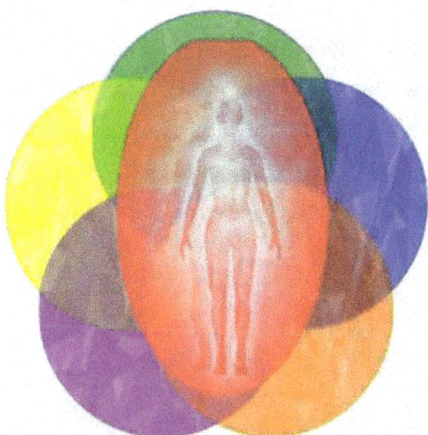

often develop an illness - such as migraine headaches, emphysema, or even arthritis.

While working on existing acute and chronic illness is essential, holistic health focuses on reaching higher levels of wellness. While the left side of the illness-wellness continuum is focused on illness and disease, the right half of the continuum invites people to constantly explore which everyday actions work for them and discover what is appropriate to move them toward maximum well-being. People are motivated by how good it feels to have lots of energy and enthusiasm for life, knowing that what they do that day will allow them to continue to feel this great for years.

Holistic health can be there for those with chronic conditions that require them to work directly with a doctor. Since holistic health focuses on the whole person, it considers all the current medications and treatments the person goes through with other health professionals and helps them implement other healthy choices that complement their current health state. Holistic health helps to bring about well-being naturally, which can lead those with chronic issues to a healthier lifestyle as well.

If you have ever wanted a more natural approach to getting rid of chronic pain, which may include:

## Conclusion

Holistic health is based on the law of nature that a whole comprises interdependent parts. The earth includes air, land, water, plants, and animals. If life and well-being are to be sustained, the elements cannot be separated, for what is happening to one is also felt by the other systems. In the same way, an individual is a whole made up of interdependent parts, which are the physical, mental, emotional, social, and spiritual. When one part is not working at its best, it impacts all of the other parts of that person.

Furthermore, this whole person, including all the parts, constantly interacts with everything in the surrounding environment. For example, when an individual is anxious about a history exam or a job interview, their nervousness may result in a physical reaction - such as a headache or a stomach ache. When people suppress anger at a parent or a boss over a long period, they

| | |
|---|---|
| Fibromyalgia | Heart Disease |
| Arthritis | Digestion Problems |
| Chronic Fatigue | Insomnia |
| Depression | Heart Disease |
| Post-accident/Surgical pain | |
| Migraines/Headaches | |
| Anxiety & Stress Issues, such as: | |
| Digestion Problems | |

109

It is time to take matters into your own hands!

*"If you change the way you look at things, the things you look at change." Wayne Dyer*

Simple and holistic living encourages the incorporation of these elements into your everyday lifestyle and awareness:

1. Diet
2. Exercise
3. Environmental measures
4. Attitude and behavior modifications
5. Relationship and spiritual counseling
6. Bioenergy enhancement

These are some of the focuses of holistic health. By definition, holistic health is about lifestyle changes, noninvasive remedies, improving the flow of a person's life-force energy, and enhancing the body's ability to heal itself.

## Holistic Living is self-empowering!

Many people opt for holistic health because it allows them to feel empowered in their health care. They don't have to be concerned about the side effects of drugs or surgery to fix them; they can take measures to enhance their well-being into their own hands.

## Knowledge is power!

*"Knowing yourself is the beginning of all wisdom." Aristotle*

Now that we have come to the end of this book, where you go from here is up to you. We recommend that you start compiling your resources, doing daily holistic health practices, and starting to make the small changes to improve your life.

## Looking for more?

Our educated and experienced team is available for you and your specific needs to help you attain the knowledge, inspiration, and guidance you need to make lasting changes for a healthier life! Check out our online platform to connect you to holistic health professionals who will help you get started on your health and healing path.

https://holisticbodyworksonline.community/

# "The journey of a thousand miles starts with a single step."
# ~Lao Tzu

# Bibliography

Andermann, A., & CLEAR Collaboration (2016). *Taking action on the social determinants of health in clinical practice: a framework for health professionals.* CMAJ: Canadian Medical Association journal = journal de l'Association medicale canadienne, 188(17-18), E474–E483. https://doi.org/10.1503/cmaj.160177

Brennan, Dan. (2021). *What to Know About Emotional Health.* WebMD. https://www.webmd.com/balance/what-to-know-about-emotional-health

Brito Sena, M., Damiano, R., Luchetti, G., & Prieto Peres, M. (2021). *Defining Spirituality in Healthcare: A Systematic Review and Conceptual Framework.* Frontiers. https://www.frontiersin.org/articles/10.3389/fpsyg.2021.756080/full

Burkhardt, Margaret & Nagai-Jacobson, Mary. (2016). *Spirituality and Health.* Nurse Key. https://nursekey.com/spirituality-and-health/

Castle Craig. (2018). *The History of Holistic Medicine.* Castle Craig. https://www.castlecraig.co.uk/therapy/history-holistic-medicine/

Division of Nutrition, Physical Activity, and Obesity. (2021). *Physical Activity Boosts Brain Health.* CDC. https://www.cdc.gov/nccdphp/dnpao/features/physical-activity-brain-health/index.html

Denton, Carolyn. (2023). *How Does Food Impact Health?* University of Minnesota. https://www.takingcharge.csh.umn.edu/how-does-food-impact-health

Department of Health. *Regular health checks.* Better Health Channel. https://www.betterhealth.vic.gov.au/health/servicesandsupport/regular-health-checks

Fuller, Kristen. (2022). *How Creating a Sense of Purpose Can Impact Your Mental Health.* Psychology Today. https://www.psychologytoday.com/us/blog/happiness-is-state-mind/202203/how-creating-sense-purpose-can-impact-your-mental-health

gomacro. (2023). *How to Start a Holistic Lifestyle.* Gomacro.com. https://www.gomacro.com/how-start-holistic-lifestyle/#:~:text=According%20to%20the%20dictionary%2C%20the,them%20all%20as%20vital%20to

Han, K. H., Hung, K. C., Cheng, Y. S., Chung, W., Sun, C. K., & Kao, C. C. (2023). *Factors affecting spiritual care competency of mental health nurses: a questionnaire-based cross-sectional study.* BMC nursing, 22(1), 202. https://doi.org/10.1186/s12912-023-01302-z

Health, Frederick. (2021). *The Connection Between Mental and Physical Health.* Frederick Health. https://www.frederickhealth.org/news/2021/october/the-connection-between-mental-and-physical-healt/

Hillyard, Debbie. (2023). *Sacred Stories/Spirits Touching CommonSpirit.* https://www.missiononline.net/sacred-stories-spirits-touching/

Holistica. (2023). *The Many Benefits of Holistic Treatments.* Holisticacare.com. https://holisticacare.com/the-many-benefits-of-holistic-treatments/

Invajy.com. (2023). *Self Improvement Blog.* Invajy.com. https://www.invajy.com/

Jasemi, M., Valizadeh, L, Zamanzadeh, V., & Keogh, B. (2017). *A Concept Analysis of Holistic Care by Hybrid Model.* Indian Journal of Palliative Care, 23(1), 71–80. https://doi.org/10.4103/0973-1075.197960

Lal, Micky. (2022). *What Are the 5 Health-Related Components of Physical Fitness?* Healthline. https://www.healthline.com/health/fitness/health-related-components-of-fitness

Lalla, J. *The Elephant Rope Parable.* The Reader's Blog. https://timesofindia.indiatimes.com/readersblog/jblblogs/the-elephants-rope-34225/

Lichtenstein, Gary. (2015). *The Importance of Sleep.* National Library of Medicine. https://www.ncbi.nlm.nih.gov/pmc/articles/PMC4849507/

Loving Life. (2021). *Physical Wellbeing & Why It's Important.* https://lovinglifeco.com/health-and-wellbeing/physical-wellbeing-why-its-important/

Madre. (2022). *5 Holistic Health Essentials And Why They Are So Important.* https://thewellco.co/the-5-aspects-of-holistic-health/

Mandolesi, L, Polverino, A., Montuori, S., Foti, F., Ferraioli, G., Sorrentino, P., & Sorrentino, G. (2018). *Effects of Physical Exercise on Cognitive Functioning and Wellbeing: Biological and Psychological Benefits.* Frontiers in Psychology, 9, 509. https://doi.org/10.3389/fpsyg.2018.00509

Makwana N. (2019). *Disaster and its impact on mental health: A narrative review.* Journal of family medicine and primary care, 8(10), 3090–3095. https://doi.org/10.4103/jfmpc.jfmpc_893_19

National Heart, Lung, and Blood Institute. (2022). *Why Is Sleep Important?* https://www.nhlbi.nih.gov/health/sleep/why-sleep-important

National Institutes of Health. (2022). *Emotional Wellness Toolkit.* NIH. https://www.nih.gov/health-information/emotional-wellness-toolkit

NCCIH. (2021). *Complementary, Alternative, or Integrative Health: What's In a Name?* NIH. https://www.nccih.nih.gov/health/complementary-alternative-or-integrative-health-whats-in-a-name

Olsson, Regan. (2021). *8 Ways to Take Care of Your Spiritual Health.* Banner Health. https://www.bannerhealth.com/healthcareblog/better-me/8-ways-to-take-care-of-your-spiritual-health

Pacheco, Danielle & Dr. Singh, Abhivav. (2023). *Why Do We Need Sleep?* Sleep Foundation. https://www.sleepfoundation.org/how-sleep-works/why-do-we-need-sleep

Peterson, T.J. (2019). *What Is Emotional Health? And How To Improve It?* HealthyPlace. https://www.healthyplace.com/other-info/mental-illness-overview/what-is-emotional-health-and-how-to-improve-it

Plumptre, Elizabeth. (2023). *The Importance of Mental Health.* VeryWellMind. https://www.verywellmind.com/the-importance-of-mental-health-for-wellbeing-5207938

Puchalski C. M. (2001). The role of spirituality in health care. Proceedings (Baylor University. Medical Center), 14(4), 352–357. https://doi.org/10.1080/08998280.2001.11927788

Reachout. *Teach your teenager coping skills for wellbeing.* Reachout. https://parents.au.reachout.com/skills-to-build/wellbeing/things-to-try-coping-skills-and-resilience/teach-your-teenager-coping-skills-for-wellbeing

Reed, Paul. (2021). *Physical Activity Is Good for the Mind and the Body.* U.S. Department of Health and Human Services. https://health.gov/news/202112/physical-activity-good-mind-and-body

Saunders J, Smith T. *Malnutrition: causes and consequences.* Clin Med (Lond). 2010 Dec; 10(6):624-7. doi: 10.7861/clinmedicine.10-6-624. PMID: 21413492; PMCID: PMC4951875.

Schulte-Körne G. (2016). *Mental Health Problems in a School Setting in Children and Adolescents.* Deutsches Arzteblatt international, 113(11), 183–190. https://doi.org/10.3238/arztebl.2016.0183

Sharma, A., Madaan, V., & Petty, F. D. (2006). *Exercise for mental health.* Primary care companion to the Journal of clinical psychiatry, 8(2), 106. https://doi.org/10.4088/pcc.v08n0208a

Shekeryk, Nick. *5 Ways managers can help employees find a sense of purpose in the workplace.* Limeade. https://www.limeade.com/resources/blog/help-employees-find-a-sense-of-purpose-in-the-workplace/

Simple Lionheart Life. (2023). *10 Benefits of Living a Simple Life.* Simple Lionheart Life. https://simplelionheartlife.com/benefits-of-a-simple-life/

Sissons, Beth. (2023). *What is emotional health and well-being?* Medical News Today. https://www.medicalnewstoday.com/articles/emotional-wellbeing

Sonia. (2020). *9 Great Benefits of Living a Simple Life.* Life's Little Pleasures and Struggles. https://www.lifespleasuresandstruggles.com/2020/09/19/9-great-benefits-of-living-a-simple-life/

Southard, M.E. (2020). *Spirituality: The Missing Link for Holistic Health Care.* American Holistic Nurses Association. https://journals.sagepub.com/doi/full/10.1177/0898010119880361 St. Catherine University. (2022). *What Is Holistic Health? Overview and Career Outcomes.* https://www.stkate.edu/healthcare-degrees/what-is-holistic-health

Stevenson, Marie. (2021). *Physical well-being and health: What it is and how to achieve it.* BetterUp. https://www.betterup.com/blog/physical-well-being-and-health-what-it-is-and-how-to-achieve-it

Templeton, Jenna. *The 8 Pillars of Holistic Health and Wellness.* Ask The Scientists. https://askthescientists.com/pillars-of-wellness/

Tewari, Aarushi. (2023). *Top 50 Wellness Quotes For A Healthier Life.* https://blog.gratefulness.me/

Thornton, Lucia. "A Brief History and Overview of Holistic Nursing." *Integrative medicine (Encinitas, Calif.)* vol. 18, 4 (2019): 32-33. https://www.ncbi.nlm.nih.gov/pmc/articles/PMC7219452/

Veazey, Karen. (2022). *Why emotional self-regulation is important and how to do it.* Medical News Today. https://www.medicalnewstoday.com/articles/emotional-self-regulation

Ventegodt, S., Kandel, I., & Merrick, J. (2007). A short history of clinical holistic medicine. *TheScientificWorldJournal*, 7, 1622–1630. https://doi.org/10.1100/tsw.2007.238.

Wein, Harrison. (2021). *Good Sleep for Good Health, Get the Rest You Need.* https://newsinhealth.nih.gov/2021/04/good-sleep-good-health

Whitman, A., DeLew, N., Chappel, A., Aysola, V., Zucherman, R., & Sommers, B. (2022). *Addressing Social Determinants of Health: Examples of Successful Evidence-Based Strategies and Current Federal Efforts.* ASPE. https://aspe.hhs.gov/sites/default/files/documents/e2b650cd64cf84aae8ff0fae7474af82/SDOH-Evidence-Review.pdf

World Health Organization. (2022). *Mental Health.* WHO. https://www.who.int/news-room/fact-sheets/detail/mental-health-strengthening-our-response

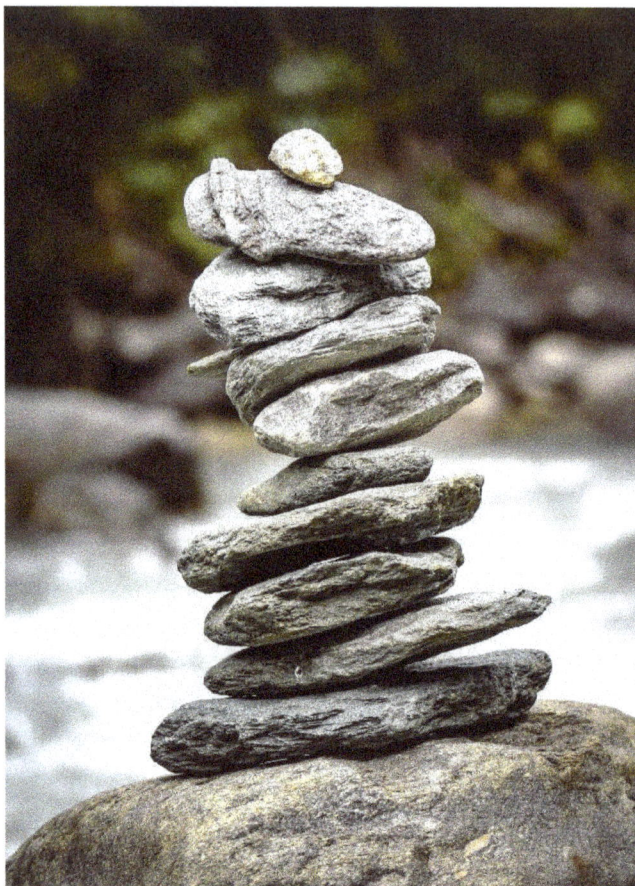

Image by Denny Franzkowiak

# Image Credits

A note about images used in this book. Every effort was made to ensure the authorized use of included images. Some of the included images are original and owned by the authors, some are from the Canva platform, others are from image sharing platforms. The Creative Commons platform, Openverse portal, ensures that marked images are in public domain or authorized for commercial use among other permissions. Pixabay allows the use of uploaded images for use under their proprietary license and all requirements have been met under that license for images found on that platform.

To view Creative Commons terms, visit:
https://creativecommons.org/publicdomain/zero/1.0/?ref=openverse
To view Pixabay's Content License Summary, visit:
https://pixabay.com/service/license-summary/

"Alpine Bird Bioblitz Volunteers" by GlacierNPS is marked with Public Domain Mark 1.0.
Child with dog image by bess.hamiti@gmail.com from Pixabay
Couple in kitchen image by Werner Heiber from Pixabay
"Elephant 1" by budz.mckenzie is marked with CC0 1.0.
"Eurasian eagle-owl" by Mathias Appel is marked with CC0 1.0.
"Forest Path" by Atraktor Studio is marked with Public Domain Mark 1.0.
"Girl biking" is marked with CC0 1.0.
"Grief" by Counseling from Pixabay
"Happy Martin Luther King Day: Holding a Jewel of meditation looking into one's own mind, Buddha statue in the lotus mudra, snow, Broadview, Seattle, Washington, USA, Saha Planet Earth, 'Tolerable' (Sanskrit Saha, 'Tolerable' as in 'barely tolerable')" by Wonderlane is marked with CC0 1.0.
Lavender image by Berkan Küçükgül from Pixabay
Old hands by Sabine van Erp from Pixabay
Stone Tower image by Denny Franzkowiak from Pixabay
"Students Run at Fort Ord" by blmcalifornia is marked with Public Domain Mark 1.0.

Author images by Stephanie Seborg – ©2023 all rights reserved
Original cover design and chapter elements by Liesl Seborg – ©2023 all rights reserved
Recipe images by Sharry Smith – ©2023 all rights reserved
Supplemental images as credited – ©2023 all rights reserved
Uncredited images – Public Domain or Canva Pro as licensed by Holistic Bodyworks, LLC

# Resources

Aetna. (2023). *Your mental health & well-being*. Aetna. https://www.aetna.com/individuals-families/mental-emotional-health.html

CARE. (2023). *Understanding mental health*. CARE. https://healthy.kaiserpermanente.org/health-wellness/mental-healthMental Health & Faith Network. (2012). Spiritual Care Network, Bridging the Gap Between Mental Health & Faith. Mental Health & Faith Network. https://www.spiritualcarenet.org/

Centers for Disease Control and Prevention. (2023). *Improving Access to Children's Mental Health Care*. https://www.cdc.gov/childrensmentalhealth/access.html

Ho, J., Funk, S., (2018) *Promoting Young Children's Social and Emotional Health*. https://www.naeyc.org/resources/pubs/yc/mar2018/promoting-social-and-emotional-health

National Institute of Mental Health. (2023). *Help for Mental Illnesses*. NIH. https://www.nimh.nih.gov/health/find-help

U.S. Department of Veterans Affairs. (2023). *V.A. mental health services*. https://www.va.gov/health-care/health-needs-conditions/mental-health/

# Acknowledgments

We both have wonderful people who have inspired us and helped us throughout the process of writing and publishing our work.

## Stephanie

First, thank you, Sharry, my coauthor, for being there for me during my healing journey and building my business (Holistic Bodyworks). You have been there for me and the company through all the growing pains of the business and long inspiration sessions with very little or no pay. With you, Holistic Bodyworks did better! I love and admire you and what you stand for personally and spiritually. You inspire me and give me the strength to keep pushing and working on my healing journey. Thank you for being you!

Second, I want to thank my staff and colleagues, who constantly remind me how important my leadership and friendship is to them. Without them, I would not have the social support I need to manifest a healing and supportive space for all of us. Thank you so much for being a part of my professional family!

Lastly, and most importantly, thank you to my family and my lovely wife for being my rock! Liesl, without you, this book would not be possible. In fact, without you, the love and passion I feel daily would not be overfilling and spilling over onto those that I help heal. I love you with every part of my being, which is powerful medicine. Thank you for all of the love and acceptance that you show me!

## Sharry

First and foremost, I thank Almighty God for making life and all things possible. Without his saving grace and healing, I would not be who and where I am today. Thank you to the doctors who "thought outside the box" and taught me how to heal myself. When my allopathic doctors dismissed me, you were there.

Thank you to Stephanie for having faith in me and allowing me to be part of your journey. I remember the days putting our heads together to create the healing environment that we share. Pay was never an issue; the love and sincere desire to help others was my reward.

Thank you to all the people who have been in my life. You played your part. To those who hurt and abused me ... I forgive you. To those who have been loving and supportive and helped me grow, I respect you.

Thank you to my ancestors who paved the way. And thank you for those to come. I will be there for you.

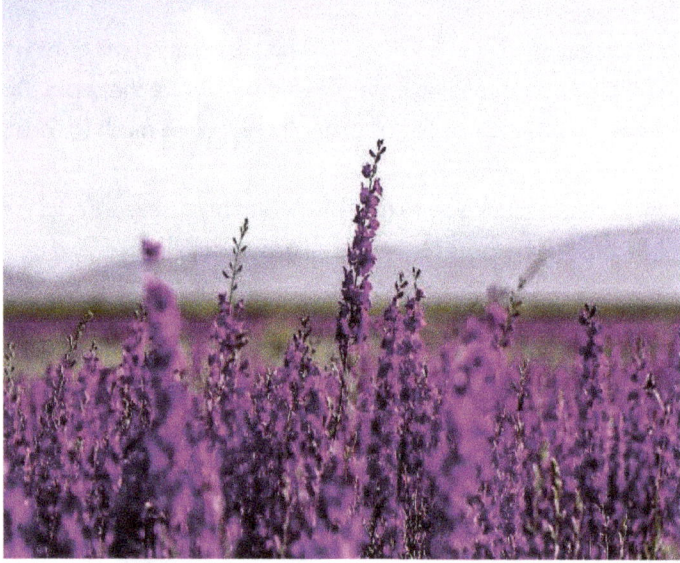

Image by Berkan Küçükgül

# About the Authors

## Stephanie Seborg

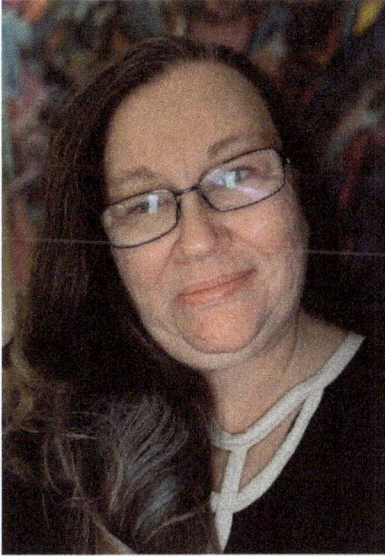

Stephanie is passionate about health and healing, which has led her to do some amazing things. She has a B.A. in Complementary and Alternative Health from Ashford University. She is a certified Reiki Master Teacher, Massage Apprentice Instructor, QHHT practitioner, Ericksonian Hypnotherapist, and Licensed Massage Therapist specializing in spiritual healing. Stephanie started diving into spiritual healing in the 90s and has been practicing and facilitating spiritual healing for others since 2005.

Her interests include reading, writing, dancing, gardening, outdoor activities (camping, hiking, fishing, etc.), helping others, natural medicine, meditation, and shamanic practices. Her main passion is to help others feel their best in all aspects of their lives, whether physical, mental, emotional, or spiritual. She loves the idea of holistic health and practicing it as well!

She is a country girl with small-town values of being a part of the community, taking care of those unable to care for themselves, and, most of all, treating everyone with kindness and respect. Although she no longer lives in the country, she still holds on to these values. And she has brought these values into her in-person business and online version of Holistic Bodyworks.

Image by Stephanie Seborg

Stephanie has worked with many holistic professionals over the years and has been actively helping others. She has brought them and others together in one place to make it easier to find holistic professionals and products that can better support the community she serves. Follow this link to check out Holistic Bodyworks Online! https://holisticbodyworksonline.community

Read More about Stephanie Here: https://holisticbodyworks.squarespace.com/blog/2018/5/27/my-personal-story-of-inspiration

## Sharry Smith

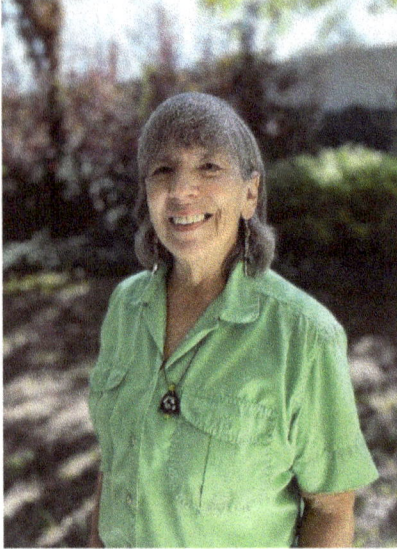

Image by Stephanie Seborg

Sharry's specialty is the John Barnes approach to Myofascial Release. After graduating from Healing Mountain Massage School, she went on to get extensive training in the John Barnes approach to Myofascial Release and continues to attend John's seminars to enhance her skills and understanding. She has used this method for several years and learned that a gentle, nurturing touch can be powerful. She also is certified in health coaching from the Dr. Sears Wellness Institute.

In her journey to become well, she learned through personal education, growth, and seeking to become the healthiest version of herself. Diving into nutrition and awareness of what her body needs, she has learned that we can take charge of our health. These ideals have helped her clients tremendously with their health and wellness.

She chose to do this work after being relieved of twelve years of chronic pain, stiffness, and limited movement. She helps guide her clients to join life again. With a passion for your best health as the foundation of her practice, she can help guide and coach you toward your best self.

She enjoys music, reading, making quilts, and tending her garden when not working. Daily yoga and Qi Gong practice, walking errands, sitting quietly, and listening to the sounds of the earth are her medicines.

Read More about Sharry Here

https://holisticbodyworks.squarespace.com/blog/2018/5/27/how-i-over-came-disability

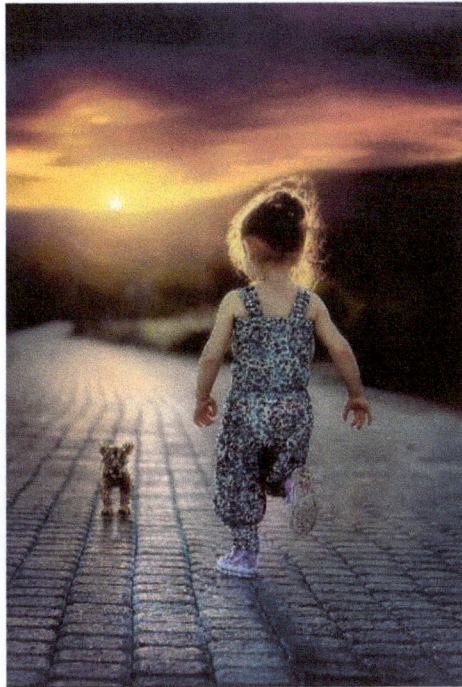

Image by bess.hamiti@gmail.com

www.ingramcontent.com/pod-product-compliance
Lightning Source LLC
Chambersburg PA
CBHW080421030426
42335CB00020B/2539